ABC of
Clinical Leadership

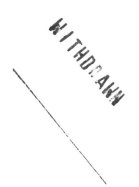

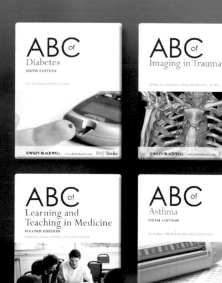
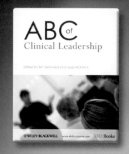
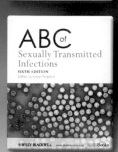

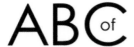

ABC of

Clinical Leadership

EDITED BY

Tim Swanwick

Director of Professional Development, London Deanery, London, UK
Visiting Professor in Medical Education, University of Bedfordshire, UK
Visiting Fellow, Institute of Education, London, UK
Honorary Senior Lecturer, Imperial College, London, UK

Judy McKimm

Associate Professor and Pro Dean, Faculty of Social and Health Sciences, Unitec, Auckland, New Zealand
Visiting Professor in Healthcare Education and Leadership, University of Bedfordshire, UK
Honorary Professor in Medical Education, Swansea University, UK
Honorary Professor in Medical Education, Oceania University of Medicine, Samoa

WILEY-BLACKWELL
A John Wiley & Sons, Ltd., Publication

BMJ|Books

This edition first published 2011, © 2011 by Blackwell Publishing Ltd

BMJ Books is an imprint of BMJ Publishing Group Limited, used under licence by Blackwell Publishing which was acquired by John Wiley & Sons in February 2007. Blackwell's publishing programme has been merged with Wiley's global Scientific, Technical and Medical business to form Wiley-Blackwell.

Registered office: John Wiley & Sons Ltd, The Atrium, Southern Gate, Chichester, West Sussex, PO19 8SQ, UK

Editorial offices: 9600 Garsington Road, Oxford, OX4 2DQ, UK

The Atrium, Southern Gate, Chichester, West Sussex, PO19 8SQ, UK

111 River Street, Hoboken, NJ 07030-5774, USA

For details of our global editorial offices, for customer services and for information about how to apply for permission to reuse the copyright material in this book please see our website at www.wiley.com/wiley-blackwell

Library of Congress Cataloging-in-Publication Data

ABC of clinical leadership / edited by Tim Swanwick, Judy McKimm.
      p. ; cm. − (ABC series)
   Includes bibliographical references and index.
   ISBN 978-1-4051-9817-2 (pbk. : alk. paper)
  1. Health services administration. 2. Health care teams – Management. 3. Physician executives. I. Swanwick, Tim. II. McKimm, Judy. III. Series: ABC series (Malden, Mass.)
   [DNLM: 1. Clinical Medicine – organization & administration – Great Britain. 2. Leadership – Great Britain. 3. Physician Executives – Great Britain. WB 102]
   RA971.A227 2011
   362.1068′3 – dc22

                                                                                        2010031704

ISBN: 9781405198172

A catalogue record for this book is available from the British Library.

Set in 9.25/12 Minion by Laserwords Private Limited, Chennai, India
Printed and bound in Malaysia by Vivar Printing Sdn Bhd
1   2011

Contents

Contributors

Beverly Alimo-Metcalfe

Professor of Leadership, Bradford University School of Management, and Real World Group, Leeds, UK

Stuart Anderson

Associate Dean of Studies, London School of Hygiene and Tropical Medicine, London, UK

Deborah Bowman

Associate Dean (Widening Participation), Senior Lecturer in Medical Ethics and Law, Centre for Medical and Healthcare Education, St George's, University of London, London, UK

Judy Butler

Senior Consultant, Coalescence Consulting Ltd, Bath, UK

Myfanwy Franks

Freelance Research Consultant, UK

Valerie Iles

Honorary Senior Lecturer, London School of Hygiene and Tropical Medicine, London, UK

Sarah Jonas

Specialty Registrar in Child and Adolescent Psychiatry, Tavistock and Portman NHS Foundation Trust, London, UK

Sir Bruce Keogh

NHS Medical Director, Department of Health, London, UK

David Kernick

General Practitioner, St Thomas Medical Group, NICE Fellow, Exeter, UK

Jennifer King

Managing Director, Edgecumbe Consulting Group Ltd, Bristol, UK

Andrew Long

Consultant Paediatrician, South London Healthcare Trust, Princess Royal University Hospital, Kent, UK

Lynn Markiewicz

Managing Director, Aston Organisation Development Ltd, Farnham, UK

Layla McCay

Specialty Registrar in General Adult Psychiatry, South London and Maudsley NHS Foundation Trust, London, UK

Judy McKimm

Associate Professor and Pro Dean, Faculty of Social and Health Sciences, Unitec, Auckland, New Zealand
Visiting Professor in Healthcare Education and Leadership, University of Bedfordshire; Honorary Professor in Medical Education, Swansea University, UK
Honorary Professor in Medical Education, Oceania University of Medicine, Samoa

Fiona Moss

Director of Medical and Dental Education, NHS London, London, UK

Tim Swanwick

Director of Professional Development, London Deanery; Visiting Professor in Medical Education, University of Bedfordshire; Visiting Fellow, Institute of Education; Honorary Senior Lecturer, Imperial College, London, UK

Michael West

Executive Dean, Aston Business School, Aston University, Birmingham, UK

Preface

The *ABC of Clinical Leadership* is designed for clinicians new to leadership and management as well as for experienced leaders. It will be relevant to doctors, dentists, nurses and other healthcare professionals at various levels, as well as to health service managers and support staff. The book is particularly appropriate for guiding doctors in training and their supervisors and trainers.

The *ABC of Clinical Leadership* has been written in the context of an increasing awareness that effective leadership is vitally important to patient care and health outcomes. Patient care is delivered by clinicians working in systems, not by individual practitioners working in isolation. To deliver healthcare effectively requires not only an understanding of those systems but also an appreciation of how to influence and improve them for the benefit of patients. This in turn requires the active participation of clinicians in leading change and improvement at all levels, from the clinical team to the department, the whole organisation and out into the wider community.

This book then aims to inform and encourage those engaged in improving clinical care, and we have been fortunate in attracting a team of authors with huge expertise and knowledge about leadership in the clinical environment. We thank them all for their contributions. What we have aimed to do is provide an introduction to some key leadership and organisational concepts as they relate to clinical practice, linking these to real-life examples and contemporary health systems. Each chapter is free-standing, although reading the whole book will provide a good grounding in clinical and healthcare leadership theory and practice. Along the way, we have provided pointers to additional resources for those who want to find out more or explore additional aspects of leadership.

The book begins with an introduction to clinical leadership, through contextualising this in key policy drivers and leadership and management theory. We move on to consider key aspects of leadership: leading teams, change, organisations and complex environments. Then we look at the specific contexts of leading clinical services and education. The later chapters consider the broad contexts of collaboration and partnership working, how gender, culture and ethical issues influence leadership and how leadership development may best be carried out. We hope that you enjoy the book, and that it stimulates you to reflect on and develop your own leadership practice and that of others.

Tim Swanwick
Judy McKimm

CHAPTER 1

The Importance of Clinical Leadership

Sarah Jonas[1], Layla McCay[2] and Sir Bruce Keogh[3]

[1]Tavistock and Portman NHS Foundation Trust, London, UK
[2]South London and Maudsley NHS Foundation Trust, London, UK
[3]Department of Health, London, UK

OVERVIEW

- Clinical leadership is vital to the success of healthcare organisations
- Good clinical leadership is associated with high-quality and cost-effective care
- Clinical leadership engages healthcare professionals in setting direction and implementing change
- Effective clinical leadership is multidisciplinary
- Clinical leadership is needed at every level

Healthcare is a huge business. Every person in the world needs it, high proportions of gross domestic product (GDP) are spent on it, governments are judged on it, populations are determined by it and almost everyone has an interest in how it is delivered. Organising and managing healthcare delivery is a complex undertaking, be it at the national level, local levels or at the level of individual interaction between healthcare professional and patient. Healthcare is usually delivered by large organisations.

In the United Kingdom, spending on healthcare accounts for 8% of GDP and the National Health Service (NHS) employs 1.4 million people, making it the third-largest civilian organisation in the world. To enable organisations of such magnitude to deliver high-quality care for all, effective leadership is vital at every level. This means having a multidisciplinary leadership and management structure which, to be truly effective, must involve all clinical professions (Figure 1.1).

What is clinical leadership?

Leadership and management are often used as overlapping concepts. However, they represent two key facets of how organisations, groups or individuals set about creating change. Leadership involves setting a vision for people, and inspiring and setting organisational values and strategic direction. Management involves directing people and resources to achieve organisational values and strategic direction established and propagated by leadership. A lack of either leadership or management makes it more difficult for an organisation to effect change or progress. Both concepts are explored in more detail in Chapters 2 and 3.

The term 'clinical leadership' is used to encapsulate the concept of clinical healthcare staff undertaking the roles of leadership: setting, inspiring and promoting values and vision, and using their clinical experience and skills to ensure the needs of the patient are the central focus in the organisation's aims and delivery. Clinical leadership is key to both promoting high-quality clinical care and transforming services to achieve higher levels of excellence. There is a role for clinical leadership at every level in healthcare organisations and systems.

Why is clinical leadership important?

Just as face-to-face patient care benefits from a multidisciplinary approach, drawing on diverse experience and skills helps achieve high-quality care at department, hospital, regional, national and international levels. As principal deliverers of healthcare, with a unique insight and expertise in healthcare need, challenges and delivery, it is clear that clinicians must be involved in leadership. Evidence shows that clinical leadership has increasingly been associated with high-performing healthcare organisations, and that effective clinical leadership in an organisation leads to both higher-quality care and greater profit.

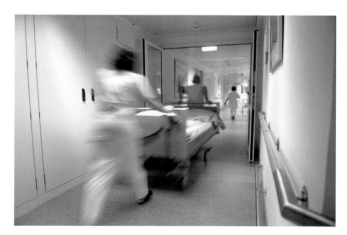

Figure 1.1 Truly effective clinical leadership is multidisciplinary. Copyright iStockphotos.

ABC of Clinical Leadership, 1st edition.
Edited by Tim Swanwick and Judy McKimm. © 2011 Blackwell Publishing Ltd.

Reviewing the NHS over the last two decades has revealed great variation in the impact of reforms across different NHS organisations, despite coherent management (non-clinical) support. Promoting and inhibiting progress and change in healthcare organisations clearly depends not only on top management but also on the level of clinical engagement in the process. The presence of effective clinical leadership is a key variable in the successful implementation and effectiveness of NHS reforms. Of particular importance is the presence of clinical champions who are willing to lead by example. This is consistent with international evidence that clinician support is critical for effective change implementation in healthcare. For this reason clinical leadership has been made central to the promotion and implementation of current and future NHS reforms, including the recent comprehensive review of the NHS on its 60th birthday.

Leadership in the NHS

When the NHS was formed in 1948, hospital management was often described as 'management by consensus', where administrative, medical and nursing hierarchies coexisted but had no power over each other. Administrators made administrative decisions, doctors made medical decisions, nurses made nursing decisions and central government made the funding decisions. Rapid increases in costs in the 1980s made this management model difficult to maintain and the government-commissioned Griffiths Report (1983) led to the introduction of general management in the NHS. This involved formalising the management arrangements, the creation of trust boards and appointing clinical directors and medical directors to manage clinical areas with the intention of aligning clinicians with the objectives of the organisation; however, this was not always achieved.

Throughout the 1990s, there arose a growing recognition that clinicians needed to be actively engaged in the leadership and management of health services in order that change might proceed unimpeded. By the next decade, it became apparent that clinical engagement was not only necessary to prevent the derailing of managerial initiatives, but a vital prerequisite to effective direction setting and change management.

Leadership and the clinical professional organisation

Since the inception of the NHS, financial power has been concentrated at the centre and clinical power has been concentrated at the periphery. However, this lack of joined-up strategic overview limits the degree of quality improvement that an organisation can undertake. International examples (Box 1.1) have shown that a joined-up approach is more likely to lead to significant quality improvement. This has led to the NHS championing clinical leadership at all levels.

Mintzberg (1992) would describe the healthcare organisation as a 'professional bureaucracy', an organisation where significant organisational decisions are made at the periphery by relatively autonomous professionals – as opposed to a 'machine bureaucracy', such as a government department, where organisational decisions are made centrally and carried out at the periphery. An essential feature of professional bureaucracies is the need for leadership to come from within the profession in order to engage that group in the vision for change. The background of a professional leader has a large impact on their effectiveness in leading and inspiring staff groups.

Box 1.1 **Case study: The US experience**

Today's growing interest in clinical leadership also derives from a number of success stories from around the world. Particularly notable are two examples from the United States, where clinicians are already actively engaged in the running of health services.

Kaiser Permanente

Kaiser Permanente is a US health management organisation where clinical leadership is central to its structure and function. Its doctors are essentially partners in the business, transcending the traditional barriers between clinicians and managers, and closely aligning priorities and strategies to create a joint mission. Clinicians are actively encouraged to take on senior management roles, and quality improvement projects are seen as internally generated rather than externally imposed.

Veterans Association

The Veterans Association (VA) is a public sector healthcare provider for US military personnel. In the 1990s, its reputation for quality care was low; it has since transformed itself into an organisation esteemed worldwide for the success of its quality improvement initiatives. These changes were led by a medical chief executive and included clinical leadership as a central premise. Today, the VA is a leader in clinical quality and has shown that clinical leadership is associated with high-quality care, and with lower-cost care.

Effective leadership in healthcare occurs at distinct levels: the strategic level, the service level and the frontline. Clinical leadership is vital to join up efforts at the different levels. As in all professional bureaucracies, a lack of effective leadership can otherwise lead to anarchy, as significant decisions involving the whole organisation can be made at the frontline with no regard for the organisation's overall strategy. Embedding clinical leadership at every level is key to ensuring that the multitude of decisions made peripherally on a daily basis in large healthcare systems add up to some concerted action aligned with the organisation's goals. When activated successfully, the professional bureaucracy will drive excellence in a way that a machine bureaucracy cannot.

Barriers to clinical engagement

Interestingly, the very qualities that make clinicians good leaders also present barriers. Historically, clinicians have been deterred from taking up leadership roles owing to the lack of remuneration, the lack of professional recognition and respect and the lack of formal training and career pathways for these roles. In particular, a culture of anti-managerialism has arisen in some organisations, where clinicians may unhelpfully refer to their clinical leader colleagues as 'going over to the dark side'. Leadership can also be perceived as a somewhat nebulous concept, and in a world of evidence-based practice, the study of leadership can be seen as non-rigorous and unscientific. It is up to clinicians to further develop the study of this vital discipline and recognise and reward the true importance and power of clinical leadership.

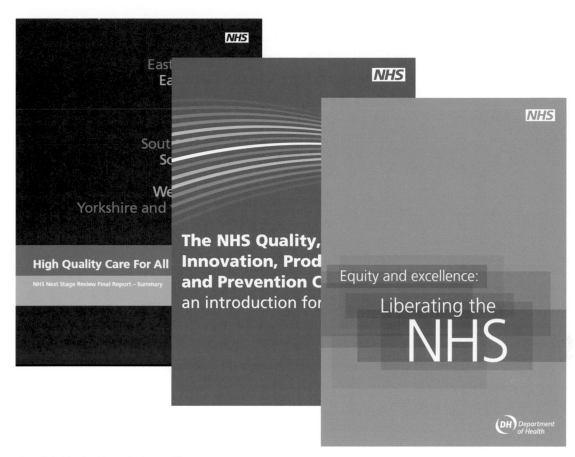

Figure 1.2 Putting clinical leadership at the heart of improvement.
Source: Department of Health, 2009; 2010.

The future of clinical leadership

In England, the publication of *High Quality Care for All* (Darzi, 2008; Department of Health, 2008) placed quality improvement at the heart of the NHS, and defined clinical leadership as an essential component of delivering improvement, setting out the role of the clinician as practitioner, partner and leader (Figure 1.2). The publication of the *Medical Leadership Competency Framework* by the Academy of Medical Royal Colleges and the NHS Institute for Innovation and Improvement (2008) and the creation of the National Leadership Council have further embedded clinical leadership as central to the future development of the NHS. A commitment that has been reiterated, in 2010, by the UK's newly elected administration (*Equity and Excellence: Liberating the NHS,* Department of Health, 2010). Throughout the world, healthcare systems are becoming increasingly expensive and the need for improving quality of care has taken centre stage. The impetus for clinical leadership to align forthcoming reforms with the needs of the patient has never been greater. The task for clinicians will be to grasp the opportunity and lead future change through effective clinical leadership.

References

Academy of Medical Royal Colleges & NHS Institute for Innovation and Improvement. *Medical Leadership Competency Framework*. NHS Institute for Innovation and Improvement, London. 2008.

Darzi A. *A High Quality Workforce: NHS Next Stage Review*. Department of Health, London. 2008.

Department of Health. *Equity and Excellence: Liberating the NHS*. The Stationery Office, London. 2010.

Department of Health. *High Quality Care for All: The NHS Next Stage Review final report*. The Stationery Office, London. 2008.

Griffiths Report. *NHS Management Inquiry*. Department of Health and Social Security, London. 1983.

McNulty T, Ferlie E. *Re-engineering Health Care: The complexities of organizational transformation*. Oxford University Press, Oxford. 2002.

Mintzberg H. *Structure in Fives: Designing effective organisations*. Prentice Hall, Harlow. 1992.

Further resources

Dickinson H, Ham C. *Engaging Doctors in Clinical Leadership: What Can We Learn from the International Experience and Research Evidence?* University of Birmingham, Birmingham. 2008.

Hamilton P, Spurgeon P, Clark J *et al*. *Engaging Doctors: Can doctors influence organisational performance? Enhancing engagement in medical leadership*. Academy of Medical Royal Colleges & NHS Institute for Innovation and Improvement, London. 2008.

Mountford J, Webb C. When clinicians lead. *The McKinsey Quarterly* **February 2009**, http://www.racma.edu.au/index.php?option=com_docman&task=doc_view&gid=573, accessed 14 July 2010.

CHAPTER 2

Leadership and Management

Andrew Long

South London Healthcare Trust, Princess Royal University Hospital, Kent, UK

> **OVERVIEW**
>
> - Management is about coping with complexity; leadership is about coping with change
> - Managers have subordinates; leaders have followers
> - Many healthcare organisations are over-managed and under-led
> - Complex organisations require good leadership and consistent management working together
> - Modern managers understand the importance of workforce needs; modern leaders recognise that successful outcomes require shared vision

Introduction

Writing in 1974, Abraham Zaleznik posed the question 'Managers and leaders: are they different?' (Zaleznik, 1974) and since then, numerous authors have attempted to both define the differences between the two activities and highlight their similarities. Managers are people that do things right' but 'leaders are people that do the right thing' is a typical distinction (Bennis & Nanus, 1985), the consensus being that management is concerned with providing order and consistency, whilst leadership is about producing change and movement (Northouse, 2004). Table 2.1 summarises the key characteristics ascribed to the activities of management and leadership.

Latterly there has been an increased resistance to the way that such analyses tend to denigrate management as somehow boring and unsatisfying. Leaders too must ensure that systems, processes and resources are in place. Furthermore, most leaders are appointed to management positions from which they are expected to lead, such as medical director within a trust or the partner responsible for quality and clinical governance in a group practice. Most recent work has taken the view that leadership is not the work of a single person but requires a multidirectional influence-relationship between leaders and followers and may therefore be seen as a collaborative endeavour. This is perhaps less true of management, where there are clear lines of accountability, power relationships and control of funding and other resources.

ABC of Clinical Leadership, 1st edition.
Edited by Tim Swanwick and Judy McKimm. © 2011 Blackwell Publishing Ltd.

The current view is a reconciliatory one. Leading and managing are distinct but complementary activities and both are important for success (Box 2.1). Indeed, the separation of the two functions – management without leadership and leadership without management – has even been argued to be harmful (Box 2.2; Figure 2.1).

> Box 2.1 **Leadership and management are both necessary for success**
>
> Leading and managing are distinct, but both are important. Organisations which are over-managed but under-led eventually lose any sense of spirit or purpose. Poorly managed organisations with strong charismatic leaders may soar temporarily only to crash shortly thereafter. The challenge of modern organisations requires the objective perspective of the manager as well as the brilliant flashes of vision and commitment wise leadership provides.
>
> *Source*: Bolman & Deal, 1997.

Table 2.1 Characteristics of management and leadership.

Aspect	Management	Leadership
Style	Transactional	Transformational
Power base	Authoritarian	Charismatic
Perspective	Short-term	Long-term
Response	Reactive	Proactive
Environment	Stability	Change
Objectives	Managing workload	Leading people
Requirements	Subordinates	Followers
Motivates through	Offering incentives	Inspiration
Needs	Objectives	Vision
Administration	Plans details	Sets direction
Decision-making	Makes decisions	Facilitates change
Desires	Results	Achievement/excellence
Risk management	Risk avoidance	Risk taking
Control	Makes rules	Breaks rules
Conflict management	Avoidance	Uses
Opportunism	Same direction	New direction
Outcomes	Takes credit	Gives credit
Blame management	Attributes blame	Takes blame
Concerned with	Being right	What is right
Motivation	Financial	Desire for excellence
Achievement	Meets targets	Finds new targets

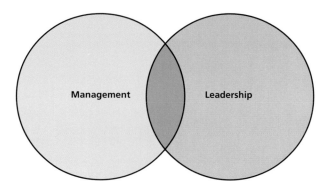

Figure 2.1 Management and leadership: Distinct but complementary activities.

Box 2.2 **The separation of management from leadership is dangerous**

[T]he separation of management from leadership is dangerous. Just as management without leadership encourages an uninspired style, which deadens activities, leadership without management encourages a disconnected style, which promotes hubris. And we all know the destructive power of hubris in organizations …

Source: Gosling & Mintzberg, 2003.

Clinicians in management

The implementation of the Griffiths Report in 1983 (Griffiths, 1983) brought about a fundamental restructuring of NHS organisation and a major reorganisation of duties and responsibilities, accountability and control. The significant increase in managers in the NHS led to a new style of organisation. Further NHS reorganisation in the 1990s recommended the 'streamlining' of management arrangements to ensure that as much of the NHS budget as possible was spent on patient care. However, it was also recognised that clinical management within organisations needed to be strengthened through the development of clinical leadership within the 'top management team' to coordinate care delivery within the organisation, to ensure greater clinical ownership of contracts with external purchasers of healthcare and to ensure that departmental budgets were managed effectively.

The role and function of doctors that took on managerial roles perceptibly changed and brought about it an inherent suspicion of any clinician who professed an interest in taking on a 'managerial' role. It was perceived, often unjustly, that there was an inherent conflict of interests, balancing expensive patient care against necessary financial savings. Consultants were slow to adapt to their autonomy being restricted through new line management relationships and this was further challenged by the introduction of a new consultant contract, which linked annual appraisal to salary benefits, introducing the concept of performance review.

Experiments with total quality management, business process re-engineering and the development and diffusion of innovation during the 1990s continued to highlight the paralysing effect on reform of 'loose coalitions of clinicians engaged in incremental

development of their own service largely on their own terms' (McNulty & Ferlie, 2002). There was a growing recognition that doctors need to be actively engaged in management and leadership of health services in order that change might proceed unimpeded.

The culmination of such thinking came in 2008 with the publication of Lord Darzi's *NHS Next Stage Review*, in which doctors, indeed all clinicians, are invited to assume the three roles of 'practitioner, partner and leader' (Darzi, 2008). The *NHS Next Stage Review* is concerned with service transformation to achieve high levels of excellence through focusing service delivery on patients' needs. The change here, though, is that it has been recognised that to re-engage clinicians to support such reforms requires not only a cultural change but also a fresh understanding of what is meant by clinical leadership.

Complex organisations

There is little doubt that the NHS, as an institution, hospitals and primary care trusts could be described as complex organisations. They are subject to many of the influences and challenges that have been experienced within the corporate business sector. The significant changes which have affected the NHS over the last 25 years have required significant adaptation on the part of both 'purchasers' and 'providers' of healthcare. It is therefore likely that concepts that work for other large organisations will have a role in allowing the component parts of the NHS to adapt to change in an equally resilient fashion. Chapters 6 and 7 examine leading and managing organisations and systems in more detail.

The work of John Kotter, Professor of Leadership at the Harvard Business School during the 1970s, identified the need for two 'distinct and complementary' systems of action, that is leadership and management to cope with increasingly complex organisations. Kotter insisted that leadership is a learnable skill that is complementary to management. His view of the US business sector at that time was that they were over-managed and under-led. In his opinion, management is all about coping with complexity in order to prevent chaos and to retain order and consistency, whereas leadership is about coping with change. With the increasing complexity of organisations, the challenges of emerging technologies, regulatory changes and market influences, it is essential that even large organisations should have the capacity to adapt. Effective leadership then, involves setting new directions, challenging assumptions and beliefs and having a broader vision.

It would seem to be equally important to keep leadership and management within the NHS in balance, and it is perceived imbalances that have on occasions led to a loss of confidence in organisations and services to manage themselves. One such case, which led to tragic and wide-reaching consequences, was the events that led up to the Bristol Inquiry (Box 2.3).

What is a manager?

Over the last 50 years, a cultural change has led to the emergence of 'the manager' as a recognised occupation. Even within the NHS, there has been a drive to attain 'management qualifications', such as an MBA, as a means of professionalising the role. Increasingly, management skills are developed and honed independent of the organisation in which the work takes place, meaning that individuals can move between private and public sector roles depending on market influences. The downside of this is that it can result in insensitivity to context and a lack of 'organisational memory', both of which are acquired through experiential learning.

Box 2.3 Case Study: Learning from Bristol (1)

A public inquiry took place to examine the management of the care of children receiving complex cardiac surgical services at the Bristol Royal Infirmary between 1984 and 1995. The inquiry was triggered by the concerns raised by a paediatric anaesthetist working within the hospital at the time who identified significant differences in outcome compared to other units undertaking a similar caseload.

The inquiry found that there were significant failings in behaviour and insight on the part of some clinicians working within the paediatric cardiac service during the period examined. It was identified that there was a lack of leadership and of teamwork. It was also perceived that the combination of circumstances that caused the deficiencies in care offered owed as much to general failings in the NHS at that time than to any individual failing. It was accepted that Bristol was in a state of transition from the 'old' NHS to the 'new' trust status. However, it was considered that it was the responsibility of senior management to devise systems that respond to problems.

The inquiry found against the chief executive of the trust for his development of a management system that applied power without clinical leadership and in which problems were neither adequately identified nor addressed. Senior managers were invited to take control but no systems existed to monitor what they did in the exercise of that control. It was a system that was over-managed and under-led.

Source: Department of Health, 2001.

Charles Handy, Visiting Professor at the London Business School, has undertaken a large body of research into organisational culture and change. He has likened the role of the manager to that of a general practitioner. He perceives that the manager is the first person to be given problems that require solutions or decisions. There is then a requirement to carry out four basic activities, which include: (i) identification of the symptoms, (ii) diagnosis of the origin of the problem, (iii) decision on the most appropriate management and (iv) commencement of the remedial process. It was his observation that often managers failed to address one of these stages, which meant that the underlying issues were not addressed and the problems returned. It is at least in part because of this that management is often seen to be about control, and creating predictable results, rather than about people.

Because managers are employed in an authority role to get things done on time and within budget, it often affects the style that they adopt to fulfil their tasks. It has been observed that many managers tend to be risk-averse and have a tendency to avoid conflict. This can make them seem rather detached from the workface and, because they generally have subordinates to perform their tasks, they may be perceived to have an authoritarian, transactional style with a keen interest in performance. They are often more interested in the fine detail that is a necessity for fulfilling the plan for the organisation.

The 'modern' manager will have an awareness of the importance of the workforce and actively promote individual and departmental development as well as an understanding of the nature of small group behaviour, role definition and the negative impact of individual stress and interdepartmental conflict. They should also have knowledge of the concepts of change management and some understanding of organisational learning theory. Once these skills are developed, the differences between leadership and management are less marked and the 'open, listening' manager who uses their power wisely and reflects on their experiences may demonstrate many skills typically associated with leadership.

Twenty-first-century leadership

Although, as highlighted in Chapter 3, the concept of leadership is a contested one, there is a developing literature examining the requirements for leadership in the twenty-first century. Joseph Rost, a retired professor from San Diego, suggests that new skill sets are required for future leaders. His definition 'Leadership is an influence relationship among leaders and followers who intend real changes that reflect their mutual purposes' reflects his view that modern generations are unlikely to accept leadership styles that have proved successful in the past. Generational changes have broken down many of the previously held hierarchical relationships and it is now accepted that not only have expectations of leaders been raised but also 'active followership' is much more important within successful organisations. This describes a dynamic relationship between follower and leader where both become committed to organisational values and the need for 'real change'. He endorses the need that the outcome of change should be the 'reflection of mutual purposes' – the understanding that drivers for change need to be developed within organisations, rather than simply responding to an externally developed set agenda.

It is generally accepted that the old 'command and control' culture, which has been prevalent in the NHS as within other complex healthcare organisations, is no longer acceptable. It is important that leaders aiming to develop the right organisational culture have a skill set that includes an emotional awareness of the needs of their employees and an understanding both of the skills required for modern communication and of the importance of work/life balance. Leaders also need to develop shared responsibility and accountability within their organisations, are responsible for the actions of managers working with them and should encourage 'followers' to ask critical questions of the organisational activities in which they are engaged.

Accountability and autonomy

In the United Kingdom, many of the changes which have been introduced within the NHS over the last two decades have been mistrusted by many employees and patient organisations as being overtly political. Public opinion still perceives the NHS to have too many managers and there is a perception that this detracts from, rather than enhances, the care of patients. If further reform is to be successful, there is a requirement for a new climate of trust to be developed.

Demands for healthcare are unpredictable and turbulent. External influences, changing populations and the nature of disease together with technological advances mean that future needs are, at the best, uncertain. As long as the NHS is perceived to be over-managed and under-led, those working within the service will be frustrated, leading to low morale and poor motivation for change. Clinical leaders need to be both accountable and transparent in their decision-making for sure, but they also need to be open to other people's points of view, to be visionary and capable of communicating that vision and motivating others to achieve their best for the benefit of patient care.

References

Bennis W, Nanus N. *Leaders: The Strategies for Taking Charge*. Harper & Row, New York. 1985.

Bolman L, Deal T. *Reframing Organizations: Artistry, Choice and Leadership*. Jossey-Bass, San Francisco. 1997.

Darzi A. *A High Quality Workforce: NHS Next Stage Review*. Department of Health, London. 2008.

Department of Health. *Learning from Bristol: The Report of the Public Inquiry into Children's Heart Surgery at the Bristol Royal Infirmary 1984–1995*. The Stationery Office, London. 2001, www.bristol-inquiry.org.uk, accessed 19 July 2010.

Gosling J, Mintzberg H. The five minds of the manager. *Harvard Business Review* 2003;**81**(11): 54–63.

Griffiths R. *NHS Management Inquiry*. Department of Health and Social Security, London. 1983.

McNulty T, Ferlie E. *Re-engineering Health Care: The Complexities of Organizational Transformation*. Oxford University Press, Oxford. 2002.

Northouse P. *Leadership: Theory and practice*, 3rd edn. Sage, London. 2004.

Zaleznik A. Managers and leaders: Are they different? *Harvard Business Review* 1974;**82**(1): 74–81.

Further resources

Adair J. *The John Adair Handbook of Leadership and Management*. Thorogood, London. 2004.

Cooper C (ed.) *Leadership and Management in the 21st Century*. Oxford University Press, Oxford. 2005.

Fullan M. *Leading in a Culture of Change*. Jossey-Bass, San Francisco. 2001.

Handy CB. *Understanding Organisations*. Penguin, London. 1993.

Kotter JP. *What Leaders Really Do*. Harvard Business School Press, Boston. 1999.

Rost JC. *Leadership for the Twenty-First Century*. Praeger, Westport, CT. 1991.

CHAPTER 3

Leadership Theories and Concepts

Tim Swanwick

London Deanery, London, UK

> **OVERVIEW**
>
> - Leadership is a social process of influence towards the attainment of a goal
> - There is no one unifying theory or framework of leadership
> - Leadership theory can be viewed as an historical progression from the attributes of the 'great man' to the leader as 'servant'
> - Leadership may also be viewed as a function of an organisation rather than of an individual
> - Leadership development requires organisational as well as individual change

'Leadership', wrote Warren Bennis and Burt Nanus 'is like the abominable snowman whose footprints are everywhere but who is nowhere to be seen' (Bennis & Nanus, 1985). But, like the abominable snowman, that hasn't stopped us trying to describe it. In this chapter we will examine the different ways in which leadership has been thought about during the course of the last century, and the relevance of those ideas to the clinical setting. We will also look at recent attempts to bind this elusive concept within the confines of that 21st century professional phenomenon, the competency framework.

In Chapter 2 we attempted to define leadership and its relationship to management. And although the nature of leadership is hotly debated, when we look through its vast literature three common themes emerge. Leadership is a process of *influence*, relating to the attainment of some sort of *goal* – which may be generally or specifically defined, such as improved partnership with patients or reducing accident and emergency department waiting times to under four hours – and it occurs in the context of a social *group*. A leader can also be defined as 'someone with followers'. Beyond that, however, it starts to get a little tricky.

A number of variables affect the way that leadership is conceived. These may be the *preoccupations of the time*, the *socio-political system* in which leadership is exercised and differences in *cultural norms and values*. So, for example, particular ways of thinking about leadership have been favoured at certain times in history; Winston Churchill was famously successful during the Second World War,

only to fail as prime minister soon afterwards. The systems in which we work affect our thinking about leadership. Favoured models in a communist or socialist state may differ from those prevalent in a free-market economy. And a raft of cultural differences influence the way the leadership is played out: individualism vs. collectivism, masculinity vs. femininity, whether leadership is seen as a far-away or nearby process, the degree to which uncertainty is tolerated and cultural orientation to the short or long term. These cultural differences are important to bear in mind when working in a multi-ethnic, multi-racial and multi-faith organisation such as the United Kingdom's National Health Service and are addressed in more depth in Chapter 12.

Trait theory

The first half of the last century saw the emergence of the idea of the 'born leader'. Trait, or 'great man', theory proposed that leaders had a number of personal qualities. You either had these qualities or you didn't; and almost invariably they seemed to be linked to a Y chromosome, perhaps reflecting the position of women in society at the time. A stroll through the wood-panelled lobbies of our Royal Colleges and Medical Schools (with the occasional notable exception) provides a painterly paean to the 'great man'. But studies in the second half of the century began to throw doubt on whether there really was a set of personal attributes that set leaders apart from the rest of the crowd, although some weakly associated generalisations – namely ability, sociability and motivation – were found. Our fascination with leadership as a set of personal attributes hasn't gone away. Daniel Goleman's recent theories of emotional intelligence (Goleman, 1996) have been highly influential and 'personal qualities' are at the heart of both the *NHS Leadership Framework* (NHS Institute for Innovation and Improvement, 2010) and the Academy of Medical Royal College's *Medical Leadership Competency Framework* (Academy of Medical Royal Colleges/NHS Institute for Innovation and Improvement, 2008). Box 3.1 lists the capabilities of emotional intelligence and their corresponding competencies.

Perhaps the most compelling evidence on personality and leadership comes from work on the 'big five' personality factors – that is the degree to which individuals exhibit extroversion, neuroticism, openness to new experience, conscientiousness and agreeableness.

ABC of Clinical Leadership, 1st edition.
Edited by Tim Swanwick and Judy McKimm. © 2011 Blackwell Publishing Ltd.

A review of the literature from across a range of sectors and contexts (Judge *et al.*, 2002) found weak but significant positive correlations with extroversion, openness to new experience and conscientiousness – leaders then tend to have personalities that lead them to do their thinking in public that make them eager to explore new ideas and to work hard. The review also found a weak but negative correlation with neuroticism, that is it helps not to be too anxious, and interestingly no link between leadership ability and agreeableness.

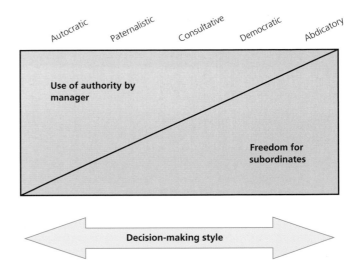

Box 3.1 **Emotional intelligence and leadership**

Self-awareness

- emotional self-awareness
- accurate self-assessment
- self-confidence

Self-management

- self-control
- trustworthiness
- conscientiousness
- adaptability
- achievement orientation
- readiness to take the initiative

Social awareness

- empathy
- organisational awareness
- service orientation

Social skill

- vision
- influence
- communication
- ability to catalyse change
- conflict management
- relationship building
- teamwork and collaboration

Figure 3.1 Spectrum of leadership decision-making styles. *Source:* After Tannenbaum & Schmidt, 1958.

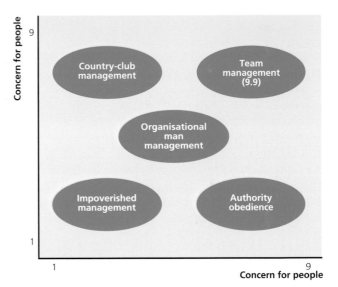

Figure 3.2 Managerial grid. *Source:* After Blake & Mouton, 1964.

Leadership styles

An alternative approach emerged in the 1940s and 1950s of leadership styles. These democratising ways of thinking about leadership focused on what the leader actually does, rather than who they were. Leadership styles theory tends to group around two issues: how *decisions* are made and where the *focus of attention* lies. A number of taxonomies of decision-making styles have appeared over the years, perhaps the most famous being that of Tannenbaum and Schmidt (1958), who describe a spectrum from the *autocratic* ('do as I say') to the *abdicatory* ('do what you like'). See Figure 3.1.

Style also relates to the extent that leadership is focused on results or the people in the organisation. Blake and Mouton's (1964) managerial grid illustrates this well with the aim being, of course, concern for the task in hand, and your staff, what they refer to as 'team management' (Figure 3.2).

Adair (1973) takes this a step further in his now famous three circles model propounding that effective leadership requires a

balance of attention not only to task and the individual but also to the team (Figure 3.3). It may be interesting to observe next time you are in the operating theatre, outpatients or a practice or departmental meeting to what extent these three areas are being looked after by those in leadership positions.

More recently, a *Harvard Business Review* article (Goleman, 2000) described six styles of leadership resulting from research on over 3500 US executives and their impact on the climate of an organisation – and that could be a hospital, a ward or a primary care trust. An authoritative style, mobilising people empathetically towards a vision, was most strongly correlated with performance.

Contingency theories

Whilst leadership styles introduced the notion that leadership could be construed as a set of behaviours, they gave little indication as to

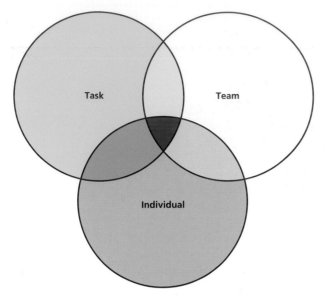

Figure 3.3 Action-centred leadership. *Source:* After Adair, 1973.

what sort of behaviours worked best in which circumstances. This was addressed most popularly by Hersey and Blanchard (1988), whose *One Minute Manager* series was a business bookstore hit. The idea that managers (or leaders) should adapt their style to the competence and commitment of their staff (or followers) is appealing and the four styles of directing, coaching, supporting and delegating can be brought into play for different people at different stages of their engagement. See Figure 3.4. So a trainee new to your practice or a nurse newly appointed to the department may require *directing* to begin with, *coaching* as their initial enthusiasm wears off, *supporting* as they develop in competence and eventually can be *delegated to* once they have developed both high 'skill' and

high 'will'. Quite often in the health service, we forget that the first three steps are important and after a brief induction junior colleagues are simply 'left to get on with it' and we are then (perhaps unreasonably) disappointed when they fail.

Transformational leadership

It became apparent in the 1980s that none of the leadership approaches to date offered advice on how to cope in environments of continual change. Models described so far were effectively transactional: followers were rewarded (or otherwise) for their efforts. Such approaches may help plan, order and organise at times of stability but, it could be argued, are inadequate for describing how people or organisations may be led through periods of significant change. A new paradigm emerged, that of *transformational leadership*, a concept best summarised under the four 'i's of Bass and Avolio (1994), namely of leaders exercising

- idealised influence;
- inspirational motivation;
- intellectual stimulation;
- individual consideration.

In the transformational model, leaders act to release human potential through the empowerment and development of followers. They paint a picture of the future and develop in followers a real sense that they want to move towards that envisioned future. Martin Luther King's 'dream' speech of 1963 is a consummate example (Luther King, 1963). Transformational leadership has proved an enduring model and has been incorporated into many public sector frameworks. Its influence can be clearly seen in 'leading people through change', 'empowering others' and 'seizing the future' of the United Kingdom's own *NHS Leadership Qualities Framework* (Figure 3.5).

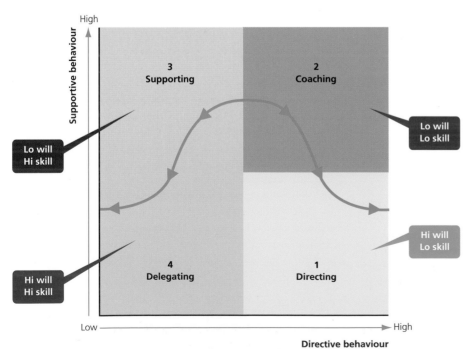

Figure 3.4 Situational leadership. *Source:* After Hersey & Blanchard, 1988.

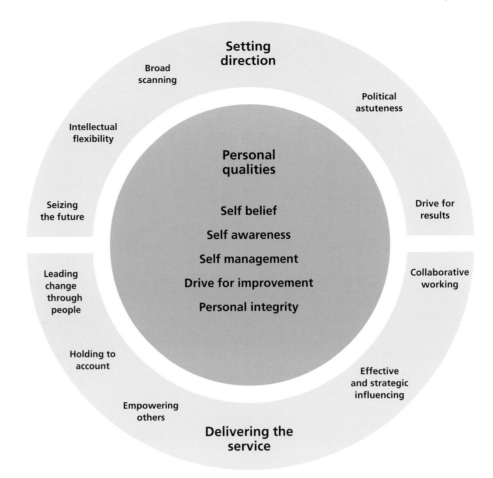

Figure 3.5 The NHS Leadership Qualities Framework. *Source:* NHS Institute for Innovation and Improvement (2010).

Charismatic leadership

One of the natural sequale of a transformational approach is the veneration of the individual leader. And in the 1980s and 1990s, charismatic leaders were flown in to turn around failing organisations and high-profile captains of industry were brought in to save health services. The charismatic leader combines a dominant personality with the self-confidence to influence others, strong role modelling and high expectations, and articulates ideological goals with strong moral overtones. Many medical leaders have also favoured the exercise of leadership in this way – the downside being that it can lead to pride, arrogance and self-obsession. The flip side of charisma is narcissism.

Servant leadership

Robert Greenleaf's (1977) idea of servant leadership provided an antidote to the bright lights of 'podium leadership' described above. Popular in the ministry, and public sector, the servant leader is said to act as a steward, appointed to serve the needs of the community which they lead, to facilitate growth and development, to persuade rather than coerce and to listen and act empathetically. Interestingly, the model also seems to translate across into the cut and thrust of a business environment, and Jim Collins' classic study of highly successful US companies *Good to Great* found that the, largely low-profile, leaders at the helm of some of the most successful US

companies combined a 'paradoxical blend of personal humility and professional will' (Collins, 2001).

Distributed leadership

We end our whistle-stop tour through the wilds of the leadership literature at 'distributed' leadership. Here, leadership is considered not to reside in one individual; it is an informal, social process where expertise is acknowledged to be distributed, boundaries to leadership are open and leadership emerges from within the connections of the organisation. This collectively embedded idea of leadership shifts the focus from the individual qualities of leaders to the process of leadership within an organisation. Leadership development then becomes not just an issue of creating more leaders but developing systems that allow leadership to be taken on by a diverse range of groups and individuals. The possibilities that open up if leadership becomes everyone's responsibility are both exciting and enabling.

Can leadership be learnt?

Posner and Kouzes (1996) assert that leadership is 'an observable, learnable set of practices', and this is certainly the assumption in the proliferation of competency frameworks such as that of the Academy of Medical Royal Colleges (Academy of Medical

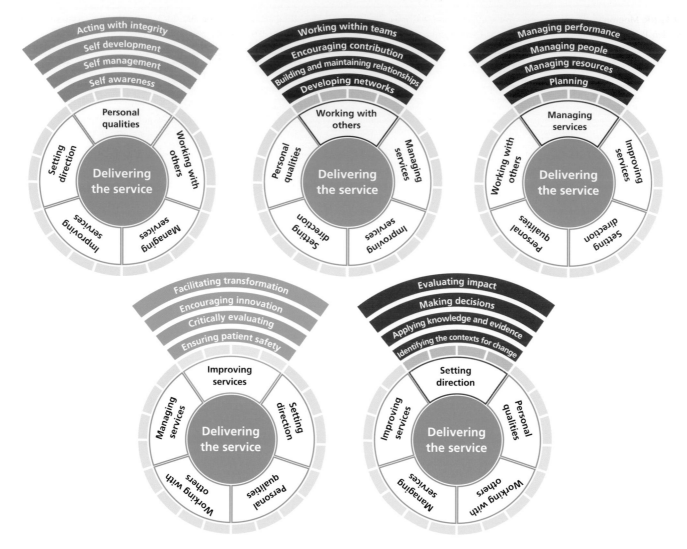

Figure 3.6 Medical Leadership Competency Framework. (a) Personal Qualities; (b) Working with Others; (c) Managing Services; (d) Improving Services; (e) Setting Direction. *Source:* Academy of Medical Royal Colleges/NHS Institute for Innovation and Improvement, 2008.

Royal Colleges/NHS Institute for Innovation and Improvement, 2008) shown in Figure 3.6. Indeed, this highlights the difference between *traits* and *competencies*, a trait being something innate or inborn, a competency, an intended and defined outcome of *learning*. But the predominant emphasis in such frameworks is on the development of the individual, and this may be at odds with our increasing awareness of the emergent and relational nature of leadership. Reading books such as this and attending leadership courses is an investment in *human capital* but in the complex and multiprofessional context of healthcare, there may also be a need to invest in *social capital*, to foster interprofessional communication and learning in the workplace and to develop cooperation within and across organisations.

What then is the role of competency frameworks? Whilst they may be of value in raising the awareness of leadership within organisations and individuals, it is in their application that issues arise and they should not be seen as a comprehensive recipe for personal or organisational success. Bolden (2004) counsels that:

they [the frameworks] should not be used to define a comprehensive set of leadership attributes, but rather to offer a 'lexicon' with which individuals, organizations, consultants and other agents can debate the nature of leadership and the associated values and relationships within their organisations.

In other words, through debating and discussing the nature of Bennis and Nanus's abominable snowman we may seek to understand both the beast, and ourselves, better.

References

Academy of Medical Royal Colleges/NHS Institute for Innovation and Improvement. *Medical Leadership Competency Framework*. NHS Institute for Innovation and Improvement, London. 2008.

Adair J. *Action-centred Leadership*. McGraw-Hill, New York. 1973.

Bass B, Avolio B. *Improving Organizational Effectiveness through Transformational Leadership*. Sage, Thousand Oaks, NJ. 1994.

Bennis W, Nanus N. *Leaders: The Strategies for Taking Charge*. Harper & Row, New York. 1985.

Blake RR, Mouton JS. *The Managerial Grid*. Gulf, Houston, TX. 1964.

Bolden R. *What is Leadership?* University of Exeter Centre for Leadership Studies, Exeter. 2004.

Collins J. *Good to Great*. Random House, London. 2001.

Goleman D. *Emotional Intelligence*. Bloomsbury, London. 1996.

Goleman D. Leadership that gets results. *Harvard Business Review* 2000;**Mar–Apr**: 78–90.

Greenleaf RK. *Servant Leadership: A Journey into the Nature of Legitimate Power and Greatness*. Paulist Press, Mahwah, NJ. 1977.

Hersey P, Blanchard K. *Management of Organizational Behaviour*. Prentice Hall, Englewood Cliffs, NJ. 1988.

Judge TA, Bono JE, Ilies R, Gerhardt MW. Personality and leadership: A qualitative and quantitative review. *Journal of Applied Psychology* **87**(4): 765–80. 2002.

Luther King M. I have a dream. 1963. http://news.bbc.co.uk/1/hi/world/americas/3170387.stm, accessed 14 July 2010.

NHS Institute for Innovation and Improvement. NHS Leadership Qualities Framework. 2010, http://www.nhsleadershipqualities.nhs.uk/assets/x/50131, accessed 22 July 2010.

Posner BZ, Kouzes JM. Ten lessons for leaders and leadership developers. *Journal of Leadership Studies* 1996;**3**(3): 3–10.

Tannenbaum R, Schmidt W. How to choose a leadership pattern: Should a leader be democratic or autocratic or something in between? *Harvard Business Review* 1958;**36**: 95–101.

Further resources

Northouse P. *Leadership: Theory and Practice*, 3rd edn. Sage, London. 2004.

CHAPTER 4

Leading Groups and Teams

Lynn Markiewicz[1] *and Michael West*[2]

[1]Aston Organisation Development Ltd, Farnham, UK
[2]Aston Business School, Aston University, Birmingham, UK

OVERVIEW

- Well-functioning multidisciplinary teams are essential to the provision of high-quality healthcare
- Clarity of leadership is a key predictor of clinical team effectiveness
- Effective leaders ensure that their teams have clear vision, objectives and effective team processes
- Team members in effective teams report high levels of role clarity, trust, safety and support
- Teams do not work in isolation: effective inter-team relationships are as important as good in-team relationships

The evidence for team-based working

A large body of research evidence identifies team working as a key predictor of success in healthcare organisations. In terms of the delivery of care, teams have been reported to reduce hospitalisation time and costs, improve service provision, enhance patient satisfaction and reduce patient mortality. In terms of staff well-being, team working is related to increased job satisfaction, reduced levels of harmful stress and increased involvement (Box 4.1) There is also evidence (World Health Organization, 2009) that effective multidisciplinary or interprofessional clinical team working is particularly related to improved quality of patient and service user care (Figure 4.1).

Box 4.1 **Benefits of team-based working: The research evidence**

- Reduced hospitalisation and associated costs
- Improved efficiency
- Improved levels of innovation in patient care
- Enhanced patient satisfaction
- Increased staff motivation and mental well-being – associated with reduced sickness absence and turnover
- Reduced error rates
- Reduced violence and aggression
- Lower patient mortality

ABC of Clinical Leadership, 1st edition.
Edited by Tim Swanwick and Judy McKimm. © 2011 Blackwell Publishing Ltd.

Why is the link so strong?

In complex organisations, where it is essential for the skills and knowledge of a number of people from different professional groups to come together to produce high-quality services, multidisciplinary teams are the vehicles for translating individual effort and skill into valued outcomes. Successful teams develop real synergy, through the contribution of all available knowledge, skills and experience to ensure the best possible decisions and outcomes. Achieving this level of team working takes time and effort but the benefits are measurable and valuable.

What is a team?

Teams come in many shapes and sizes and it is often a challenge to clearly define the boundaries of healthcare teams, which can seem

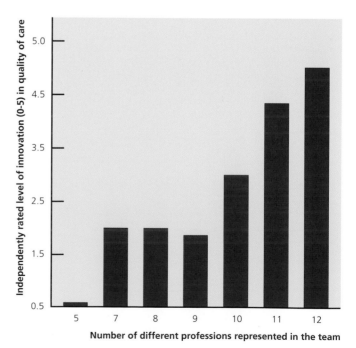

Figure 4.1 Healthcare team innovation.
Professionally diverse teams have been found to be more innovative than uni-disciplinary teams. Innovations introduced by such teams were also found to be more radical and to have significantly more impact on patient care. *Source*: Borrill *et al.*, 2000.

to stretch into other services and include different professionals who spend relatively more or less time in the team. A practical definition of a team is:

a group of people who have clear shared objectives, who need to work interdependently to achieve these objectives and who are able to regularly take time to review the way in which the team is working to achieve those objectives.

It is rare these days to find individuals who work in only one team. This can lead to confusion over individual priorities and objectives; so it is essential that all team members have a clear understanding of their role in each of the teams in which they work. One of these will usually be what could be regarded as their 'home team', that is the team whose objectives influence the way they work in all the other teams in which they are involved. In complex organisations, the ability to identify individual teams is important, but equally important is the need to map 'team communities'. Teams do not exist in isolation; they can only succeed when they work effectively with other relevant teams, for example the teams that make up a patient pathway (Figure 4.2).

Key dimensions of effective clinical teams

Effective clinical teams demonstrate a number of key features, including clarity of identity, team objectives, role clarity and effective team and inter-team processes (Box 4.2).

Box 4.2 **Characteristics of effective teams**

- Clear team identity
- Clear team objectives
- Role clarity
- Effective team processes
  - decision-making
  - communication
  - constructive debate
- Effective inter-team working
- Clarity of leadership

Team identity

Team identity is important for a number of reasons:

- Humans are social beings who need to relate to those around them. Strong team identity provides the feelings of safety and support that enable individuals to do their best work.
- Team identity provides clarity of purpose and direction for the work of team members.
- Team identity enables organisations to order work in ways that reduce duplication of effort and enhance synergy.
- Task identity has been found to contribute to satisfaction of intrinsic individual needs and therefore influences a variety of useful outcomes, such as reduced absenteeism, increased work motivation and high-quality work performance.

A key task for team leaders is to enable the development of a clear team identity which is related to the organisation's overall purpose.

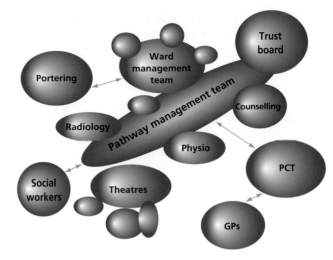

Figure 4.2 Team communities.
Team communities bring together a number of teams which rely on each other to a greater or lesser extent to deliver higher-level outcomes.

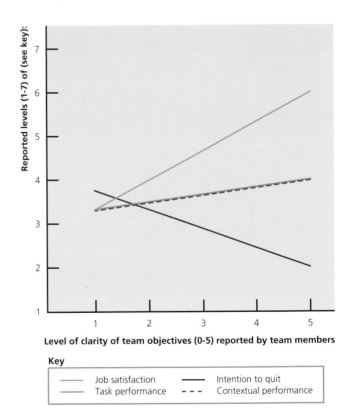

Figure 4.3 Clarity of objectives: effects.
Clarity of objectives has a number of desirable effects. Data from 61 acute trusts in England.

Team objectives

The reason why people are organised to work in teams is to achieve a common goal or purpose that will be achieved more successfully if they work together rather than individually. This notion of shared purpose is a defining feature of teams at work. Research shows that clarity of objectives is closely related to levels of individual job satisfaction, intention to quit and to task and contextual performance (Figure 4.3).

Effective team objectives describe the specific outcomes by which success will be measured, that is the results, consequences, products or impacts of actions taken by team members. These objectives also need to

- have an obvious fit with the organisation's purpose and objectives;
- be few enough to provide focus on what is most important (the most effective teams have been found to have between six and eight objectives);
- have the committed support of the next level of management and of other teams which can influence the achievement of the team's objectives.

Role clarity

Teams are created to enable people with different knowledge, skills and experience to come together to create synergy. All too often, however, lack of role clarity leads to the duplication of effort or gaps in communication and service provision. Such difficulties increase levels of distrust, decrease respect between team colleagues and increase levels of harmful conflict.

Role clarity and mutual understanding of roles amongst team members is essential for the creation of synergy. There is evidence also that role clarity increases team member confidence and job satisfaction.

Effective team processes

Decision-making

One of the principles underlying team-based working as a way of structuring and managing organisations is that teams make better decisions than individuals do.

In well-functioning teams, individuals who have relevant knowledge and experience are able to influence decisions and willingly do so. This does not mean that everyone is included in all decisions, but that team members are clear about who is involved in what type of decision and agree with the criteria for involvement. Effective teams regularly review involvement in different types of decisions to ensure that all relevant team members are involved.

Team leaders need also to be aware of the social processes which can undermine the effectiveness of team decision-making and to structure discussions in ways that ensure that all available knowledge and experience is utilised (Box 4.3).

Box 4.3 **Factors which undermine effective decision-making**

- Personality factors – e.g. knowledgeable team members may not contribute because of shyness
- Social conformity – individuals may withhold opinions or information which appears to be contrary to the majority view
- Skills – those who have excellent presentation skills may unduly influence others in the team
- Individual dominance – 'air time' and expertise are correlated in high-performing teams and uncorrelated in poorly performing teams
- Status and hierarchy – more senior members of the team may have an undue influence and may inhibit others from contributing their views

---

Communication

Effective communication takes place when each team member receives all of the information they require to carry out their job role and has access to information that will challenge them to think about and adapt their role and ways of working.

Effective team communication requires a climate of participative safety, sufficient team member interaction and effective information exchange.

Participative safety

Effective teams are places where every team member feels safe to express her/his views, ask for help or advice and is confident to put forward new ideas and suggestions about changes to the way the team is working. This will enable individuals to take appropriate risks, which are necessary for the development of creativity and innovation. Trust takes time to develop and needs to be continually nurtured. Effective leaders model appropriate behaviours and put in place processes which enable trust and respect between team members to develop (Box 4.4).

Box 4.4 **To develop trust in teams**

- Provide opportunities for team members to discuss values and aspirations
- Highlight interdependency of outcomes
- Ensure role clarity and good information flow
- Encourage team members to take appropriate risks
- Talk positively about team members and others outside of the team

---

Interaction

Research (Borrill *et al.*, 2000) shows that those teams that have regular meetings also report higher levels of innovation (Figure 4.4). It is therefore necessary to have well-managed, whole-team meetings with some regularity. This can be a challenge, particularly in busy and geographically dispersed teams where team members may see each other very infrequently. However, the potential costs of not meeting often enough are high. Leaders therefore need to explore different ways of ensuring sufficient team member interaction.

Information sharing

Information is not only crucial to the effective achievement of team tasks; it is also a source of power. Distrust within teams often arises because people feel that information has been withheld or used in a manipulative way. It is essential for teams to regularly check that all team members feel they are receiving the information they need and that it is easily accessible. Often a review will, in itself, allay fears about lack of access to information.

Constructive debate

Constructive debate is necessary in teams to ensure high-quality outcomes and to prompt a constant flow of innovation in care or service development and in ways of working. It also fosters independent thinking and professional development amongst team members and encourages the creation of strong team identity and

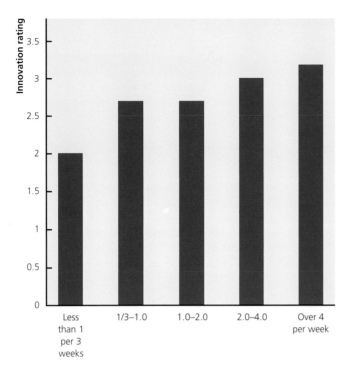

Figure 4.4 Meeting frequency.
In primary healthcare teams, regular meetings are associated with greater levels of innovation; teams which had at least one meeting a week were judged by external raters to have introduced a greater number of innovations, and innovations which were of a greater magnitude. *Source*: Borrill *et al.*, 2000.

team member attachment. This is the very opposite of the consequences of interpersonal conflict in teams. Where there are high levels of interpersonal conflict, there are often low levels of achievement, high levels of employee stress and very little innovation or personal development. Effective team leaders establish and maintain a climate of constructive debate in the team and with other relevant teams (Box 4.5 and Box 4.6).

Box 4.5 **Team climate for constructive debate**

- Openness to and exploration of opposing opinions
- Concern for quality and innovation
- Tolerance of diversity
- Concern for the integration of ideas

Box 4.6 **Case study: Effective team leadership**

A new head of department, Jane, has been appointed to the older adults' service team. After three months, many team members are complaining about the 'dictatorial' approach of the new head. They say that decisions are made without consultation, they are emailed about 'rules' and feel that they are not being treated or consulted as expert health professionals with a wealth of experience in the field. Two members of the team go off sick; others feel as if they want to leave. This comes to a head when two members of the team approach the senior management about their concerns.

Jane's line manager talks both with Jane and with the team and attends two team meetings as an observer. As a result, a coach is appointed to work with Jane to help her develop a more constructive team climate. Regular team meetings are established, information is shared more openly and Jane is reminded to speak with people as well as email them. Key objectives are agreed and developed through a departmental plan and different team members are invited to lead on specific initiatives. After six months, the team reports working in a much more collegial, trustful and functional way and Jane herself is feeling much more in control through having the support of the team.

Inter-team working

The ability of teams to form effective cooperative relationships with other teams is as important to success as the ability of team colleagues to work effectively together. Team leaders need to help their colleagues to identify relevant partner or inter-team relationships and to ensure that these flourish through

- acknowledged mutual benefit;
- partner role clarity;
- understanding about and respect for different ways of working;
- shared commitment to high-quality outcomes;
- interprofessional trust and respect.

Clarity of leadership

Traditionally in healthcare organisations there has been a lack of clarity about team leadership and yet research shows (West *et al.*,

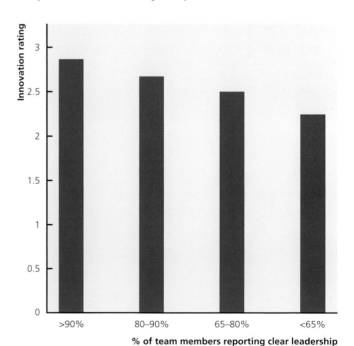

Figure 4.5 Leadership and team effectiveness.
Leadership clarity is associated with improved team effectiveness and particularly with clear team objectives, high levels of participation, commitment to excellence and support for innovation.
Source: West *et al.*, 2003.

2003) that clarity of leadership is correlated with the amount of effective team working, with levels of stress amongst team members and with levels of team innovation (Figure 4.5).

It is necessary, therefore, for team leaders to regularly discuss and review the nature of their leadership role with team members. This will include discussion about responsibilities for

- decision-making;
- managing team processes;
- supporting team and team member development.

The role of clinical team leadership is often challenging, but teams simply cannot achieve their full potential without clear and effective leadership. Part of this is ensuring that all team members understand who the team leader is and what exactly that role entails in a specific team.

References

Borrill CS, Carletta J, Carter AJ *et al. The Effectiveness of Health Care Teams in the NHS*. Department of Health, London. 2000.

West MA, Borrill CS, Dawson JF *et al.* Leadership clarity and team innovation in health care. *Leadership Quarterly* 2003;**14**: 393–410.

World Health Organization. *Framework for Action on Interprofessional Education and Collaborative Practice*. WHO, Geneva. 2009.

Further resources

Jelphs K, Dickinson H. *Working in Teams*. Policy Press, London. 2008.

West MA. *Effective Teamwork: Practical Lessons from Organisational Research*, 2nd edn. Blackwell Publishing, London. 2004.

West MA, Markiewicz L. *Building Team-based Working: A Practical Guide to Organisational Transformation*. BPS Blackwell, Oxford. 2004.

A range of research papers and diagnostic and development materials relating to team based working can be found at www.astonod.com.

CHAPTER 5

Leading and Managing Change

Valerie Iles

London School of Hygiene and Tropical Medicine, London, UK

> **OVERVIEW**
>
> • Change may be described as planned, emergent or spontaneous
>
> • Approaches to leading and managing change need to fit the context, organisation or system
>
> • Contexts for change fit into four domains: the known, the knowable, the complex and the chaotic, each of which require different approaches
>
> • Behaviour is as important as techniques when managing change
>
> • Effective leadership behaviours for managing change involve caring, conversations, respect and authenticity

Introduction

There is no single 'best' way of delivering change. The approach you choose should depend on the nature of the change, the people and professions involved and the context. In this chapter we focus on some fundamental principles of leading and managing change.

Three schools of change

In this chapter we will consider three main types of change: planned, emergent and spontaneous.

Planned change

An initial analysis leads to a change agenda, an action plan and an implementation programme. On completion the change is subject to review or evaluation. See Figure 5.1.

Emergent change

Here, change leaders work with people from an organisation who have 'authenticity and intuition' with which they understand and view the organisation. Patterns of behaviour that indicate the direction of change already underway are identified and encouraged. Whereas planned change works entirely with explicit knowledge, emergent change also involves tacit knowledge.

Spontaneous change

Where systems are largely self-organising, interventions from the outside often lead to unintended consequences or are defeated by the re-emergence of existing dynamics. Here change leaders concentrate on the relationships between elements within the system (e.g. people), focusing on behaviours rather than analysis or narrative.

Different contexts for change

The context for change provides insight into which approach might be used. Mark and Snowden (2006) identify four 'innovation epistemologies', each benefiting from different research methods and leadership styles. They suggest that we can engage with innovation and change in four different domains:

• the known;
• the knowable;
• the complex;
• the chaotic.

The known

Here, there are clear cause-and-effect relationships: A causes B. If we want to achieve B then we can do A, and we can undertake research to check that A is better than X or Y at achieving B. In the domain of the known, leaders need to ensure effective ways of sensing incoming data, categorising it and responding with predictive models in accordance with best practice (Box 5.1). The

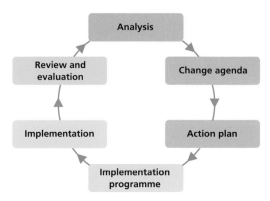

Figure 5.1 Planned change.

ABC of Clinical Leadership, 1st edition.
Edited by Tim Swanwick and Judy McKimm. © 2011 Blackwell Publishing Ltd.

leadership style can be called 'feudal': 'this is the best way of doing things, so this is what we must all do' (Mark & Snowden, 2006).

Box 5.1 **Case study: Researching the 'known'**

The hospital's clinical lead for diabetic care is asked to consider trialling a new drug designed to modulate peaks and troughs in blood sugar levels in patients using a particular insulin regime. She agrees to be involved in a randomised controlled trial to explore whether the new drug is better than the previous regime at keeping the patients' diabetes stable.

The knowable

Cause and effect relationships also exist here, but are less clear, perhaps because there is some distance between them in time or place. The relationships may only be known to a few experts. Research methods include experiment, fact-finding and scenario planning, aiming to elucidate the cause-and-effect relationships more clearly. Leadership here is 'oligarchic', held by the small number of informed individuals who understand the challenges (Box 5.2).

Box 5.2 **Case study: Exploring the 'knowable'**

The local primary care trust identifies that an increasing number of women are choosing to have home births through the new community midwife-led service. Whilst the team welcome women's right to choose the place of birth, some concerns have been expressed that there is a link between this emerging trend and the recent increase in admissions to the special care baby unit (SCBU). The team decide to carry out research with the medical and health professionals involved in both services including interviews and data analysis of maternal admission rates and SCBU admissions.

The complex

This domain contains discernible patterns (which help us understand problems) and cause-and-effect relationships. The number of agents and the frequency, richness and unpredictability of their interactions mean that patterns can be perceived but not easily categorised or predicted. Research methods relevant to the knowable and known domains are inappropriate and can be misleading: suggesting causality where there is none, based on coherence apparent only in retrospect. A wide range of (possibly innovative and less conventional) research methods need to be used. The most effective leadership style is 'emergent': which combines effective administrative procedures and safe governance with an enabling and adaptive approach (Box 5.3).

The chaotic

In this domain there are no perceivable relationships. The system is too turbulent, and time to investigate change is not available. Here, a leader needs to be able to act quickly through a hierarchy where decisions can be relayed quickly and acted upon without question.

Authority is required to 'control' the space so as to move it into the knowable, the known or the complex (Box 5.4).

Box 5.3 **Case study: Engaging with the 'complex'**

Following a series of complaints about the professional attitudes and behaviour of staff, the hospital medical director decides that there is a need to attend to professionalism within the organisation. A trust-wide series of meetings is established to focus on the issue to explore what staff understand about their professional roles, responsibilities and relationships. There is no sense as to what may emerge from the process but, over a period of a year, complaints begin to fall and there is a noticeable change in the culture of the organisation.

Box 5.4 **Case study: Managing chaos**

The accident and emergency department at the largest hospital in the area has a plan for dealing with major incidents. A train derails two miles from the hospital with over 200 people killed or injured. Emergency staff are initially overwhelmed by the scale of the disaster. However, rapid and collaborative action by hospital managers, senior clinicians and the ambulance service in accordance with the plan leads to mobilisation of key staff to the scene. The injured are rapidly triaged and taken to the most appropriate centres in the area; only the most seriously injured are brought to the major hospital. Prompt and assertive action quickly brings the 'chaotic' into the 'knowable' and the 'known'.

Where a change is wholly 'known' in nature (i.e. it is clear that an alternative way of working yields better outcomes), a planned approach is appropriate. Where the nature of the change is knowable, the emergent approach may be better, and with complex change the spontaneous approach should be chosen. Most situations in healthcare are complex and do not fall neatly into one of these domains, especially that of the 'known'. Change leaders need to use all three approaches to change simultaneously and not rely primarily on explicit planned change methods such as those shown in Figure 5.1. Chapter 7 further discusses complexity.

Table 5.1 depicts a matrix of approaches to managing planned, emergent or spontaneous change. Leading change effectively requires the rigorous, competent and creative use of all boxes in the matrix. In practice, however, it is often the case that

- Individual change leaders prefer one approach and undervalue the others. So a conversation that unearths assumptions and judgements can allow a team of people with different preferences to work together more effectively.
- Instead of creative competence in each of the 'boxes' an unaware combination is used. Clear thinking about each of the boxes in turn can prevent this.
- Reflection is usually forgotten, so very little experiential learning takes place about how to lead change effectively. Although time for reflection is difficult to find, it is a very worthwhile investment – as

Table 5.1 Approaches to change.

	Planned or deliberate change: analysis followed by plan and implementation	Spontaneous change: events, actions and behaviours emerge spontaneously from interactions in a complex adaptive system	Emergent change: foster, craft, discover things, detect patterns
Prospective *Thinking ahead*	Undertake a rigorous analysis that leads to a list of critical issues that need to be addressed, and some form of implementation programme.	Engage with a wide range of people, encouraging them to contribute their perspective and to take responsibility for playing their part in shaping the analysis and the design.	Work with the people with 'tacit knowledge', authentic and intuitive understanding of the organisation. Experiment with different ideas and look for patterns in the experience of the organisation.
	Key skills: analytical and computational	*Key skills:* listening, being comfortable with ambiguity	*Key skills:* spotting patterns, identifying authenticity
Real time *Implementing*	Manage the programme or project, using sound, proven methods for monitoring progress.	Keep in mind, and voice for others, the spirit of the programme of change; help others to behave in the spirit of this plan.	Make all your usual everyday decisions that appear to have little connection with the implementation plan. Take opportunities as they arise, fostering and crafting choices to make the best of each unforeseen situation. Interpret all sorts of knowledge and information, tacit as well as explicit, and bring meaning to events as they unfurl.
	Language used: critical path, compliance, milestones, progress reports, contingency plans, performance management	*Attributes needed:* dynamic poise, attentiveness, flexibility and responsiveness	
Retrospective *Reflecting*	Compare actual events and outcomes with those of the plan, and with the analysis that led to the plan. In practice, this can have a developmental intent (enabling better analysis and planning in the future) or a judgemental one (performance management).	Try to understand what actually happened and how, by considering the events and processes, behaviours and relationships emerged as time went on. This gives a better understanding of the dynamics of the system and enables the design of development programmes that will influence the way people respond in the future.	Tell stories: help people make sense of what has happened, by selecting some events and decisions and not others. Stories woven here are not accurate pictures of reality but simplified, coherent versions of reality that can be told to multiple stakeholders. This engenders a sense of meaning and of belonging to a longer narrative, which can become part of the history of the service or organisation.
		Tools used: facilitated reflection, informal reflection, non-blame feedback, systems thinking	

long as it is conducted with the aim of understanding rather than seeking to apportion blame.

The planned, 'linear' model of change dominates even in contexts where it is the least useful. This tendency is difficult to counter and change leaders need to be able to use the language of the planned alongside other approaches to shift the thinking of those who are unfamiliar or uncomfortable with less certain approaches.

Behaviours when leading change

The effective change leader requires a toolkit of appropriate actions, analyses and competences; however, less is spoken about leadership behaviours and values and we therefore turn to these next.

The need to care

If we are to effect beneficial change in patients and in organisations, we are more likely to do so if we care about the growth and development of others. This requires acts of work and courage. Acts of work can include gathering data, finding out about the interests,

enthusiasms and personalities of staff involved and meeting with all of them. Acts of courage could be discussing the change with people who see little need for it, finding out the views of others about existing problems and being prepared to challenge and change your own solutions and approaches.

In any situation, it is useful to ask:

- Did I care enough here?
- Did I do as much work as was needed?
- Was I sufficiently courageous?

Concentrating on the simple hard at the expense of the complicated easy

Imagine we banned the term 'communication' and did not think about a 'communication strategy'. We would be forced instead to think about

- Who needs to hear what, and from whom?
- Who needs to say what, and to whom?
- Who needs to ask what, and of whom?
- Who needs to discuss what, and with whom?

This calls upon different kinds of action and energy from that of 'developing and implementing a communication strategy'? This is an example of focusing on the *simple* hard instead of the *complicated* easy.

The *simple* requires clear but straightforward thinking about what needs to be done, some careful thought about how to do it and courage to carry it out. The *complicated*, like writing that communication strategy, calls upon much more of our intellect, but little else. While the *complicated* often involves an analysis, or a computation that can be considered to yield a 'right' answer, the *simple* is indeed hard, and, although we will never get it right, we will get less bad at it with practice. We can take pleasure in learning and growing as we do. While some *complicated* stuff is needed, it is the *simple* that determines success. And often that comes down simply to 'conversation'.

Conversation as the vehicle for change

Simple, empathic, purposeful, ongoing conversations are the essence of good management. They may be opportunistic and informal or planned and formal. The important thing is to bring together people's needs, enthusiasms and aspirations with the needs and ambitions of the organisation. The outcome comprises three rules of good management:

- a set of shared expectations about what will be done and how;
- a mutual confidence that there are the skills and resources to achieve it
- ongoing feedback on how things are going.

Change arises as a result of multiple, authentic conversations over time, most of which will be unrehearsed and emergent.

Respectful uncertainty

Perhaps the most valuable stance to take when considering change is that of respectful uncertainty: constantly looking at a system with a degree of creative suspicion. Not challenging for the sake of it, yet not leaving things as they are because of assurances from those involved that all is well. Being respectful of the people involved, their intentions and the practices they have developed is vital. However, at the same time, a change leader needs to gently challenge any certainty that these are best or only ways, and demonstrate confidence in people's ability and willingness to consider other options.

Bringing choices into awareness

We all develop routines to help us deal with the world. However, we could not function if conscious choices had to be made about options open to us every moment of the day. Many choices therefore operate on a subconscious level. Some change requires people to do differently things that they are currently doing on autopilot.

Awareness of people's emotional responses to change (Figure 5.2) can help a change leader to respond and support people appropriately. If change leaders use a heavy-handed, coercive approach,

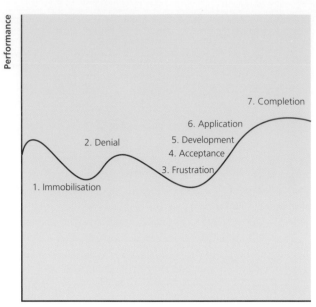

Figure 5.2 Emotional responses to change. *Source*: Adapted from Hay, 1996.

motivation and goodwill can be damaged. A lighter touch, involving gentle querying about activities and refreshing ambitions, can remind people of certain decisions and promote openness to change.

Speaking to what matters to others

Above all when engaging with others, we must speak to what matters to them. If we treat the healthcare context as a marketplace and simply advocate efficient transactions, we may achieve a valuable amount of systematisation and reduce undue variation in practice and in outcomes. But we will also alienate people who see healthcare as something more: something with elements of the 'gift economy' in which there is a covenant between care giver and care receiver.

Effective change leaders will encourage and demonstrate both sets of care behaviours (Table 5.2).

Behaving like you

When leading change, integrity is more important than heroism. So, while change leaders may want to move outside their comfort

Table 5.2 Transactional care and the 'gift economy'.

Care as a set of marketplace transactions	Care with elements of the gift economy
Patient or service cared for	Patient or service cared about
Focus on objectivity, activities that can be measured and counted	Acceptance of the importance of subjective judgement, wisdom and silence
Healthcare professionals and services seen as de-personalised units of production	The meaning of an encounter for both patient and healthcare professional is seen as important

zones to develop new skills, they must always feel in harmony with others. In particular

- Find gentle ways of saying hard things, then you will say them.
- Divide tasks into do-able chunks.
- Look for allies, people who will support *and* challenge you.

Conclusion

Leading change involves a range of skills and behaviours, many of which can be learnt. In this chapter, we have looked at the management of change through two lenses: change as planned, emergent or spontaneous and in terms of four domains or contexts for innovation. Most importantly, we have emphasised that an effective change leader needs to lead by example, through appropriate, authentic behaviours, always making the link between care and change.

Only lead change when you care, and when you do care, find ways of leading change.

References

Hay J. *Transactional Analysis for Trainers*. Sherwood Publishing, Watford. 1996.

Mark A, Snowden D. Researching practice or practising research: Innovating methods in health care: The contribution of Cynefin. In: A Casebeer, A Harrison, A Mark (eds), *Innovations in Health Care*. Palgrave Macmillan, Basingstoke. 2006.

Further resources

Iles V. *Really Managing Heath Care*. Open University Press, Milton Keynes. 2005.

Iles V, Cranfield S. *Developing Change Management Skills*. SDO, London. 2004.

Mintzberg H, Ghoshal S. *The Strategy Process: Global Edition: Concepts, Contexts, Cases*. Prentice Hall, Harlow. 2002.

CHAPTER 6

Leading Organisations

Stuart Anderson

London School of Hygiene and Tropical Medicine, London, UK

> **OVERVIEW**
>
> - Leading organisations requires an understanding of how departments run and how they relate to each other
> - Leadership plays a crucial part in shaping and changing the organisation's culture
> - Flexibility in organisational structures is essential to ensure best fit to local contexts
> - Clinical leaders need to be aware of the different sources of their power and to know which form to exercise when
> - The key organisational resource is its people, and the development of both human and social capital is important for organisational effectiveness

Organisational dimensions

The introduction to the *British Medical Journal*'s 2009 debate on leadership declared that clinical leaders 'must understand the big picture along with its component elements as well as their own position in it and how they influence it' (Imison & Giordano, 2009). This chapter describes clinical leadership at the organisational level.

Healthcare organisations vary greatly in size, purpose and complexity. Organisations can be conceptualised in many ways, with different theories emphasising institutions, resources or the environment. Metaphors used to describe them include machines, cultures and organisms.

Many models have been developed to help conceptualise the component parts of organisations and how they interact. The Burke-Litwin Model (Figure 6.1) (1991) presents a framework using an open systems approach that provides a helpful way of thinking about how leadership relates to the functioning of the organisation overall.

The model flows from top to bottom. Dimensions in the top half (external environment, mission and strategy, culture and leadership) constitute the transformational factors, those that bring about change in the whole organisation. Dimensions in the bottom half are transactional factors, those concerned with day-to-day operations.

The external environment at the top provides the inputs to the organisation; individual and organisational performance at the bottom are the outputs; the boxes in between constitute the key elements of transformation. Whilst effective leadership is the key to achieving change in transformational factors, change in transactional factors is achieved by managers focusing on improvement. Leaders must thus retain a firm grip on management practices.

This chapter focuses on those factors with which the leader needs to engage directly, as indicated by the arrows in the model. The model indicates that leaders need to engage not only with the transformational factors but also with transactional factors such as structure, management practices and systems. A good knowledge and understanding of these dimensions is needed if leaders are to ensure the optimal functioning of their organisations.

External environment

This refers to those aspects of the external social, political and economic climate that have an impact on organisational performance. It covers everything from current political priorities and changes in legislation to economic constraints on health services and health scares reported in the media. Clinical leaders have little control over the external environment, but they can sometimes anticipate it and they can make sure that whatever resources are available are used efficiently and effectively.

An understanding of the effective use of clinical resources involves not simply recognising what resources are used in healthcare but understanding all of its inputs. Black and Gruen (2005) describe these as

- medical knowledge and its application;
- medical paradigms (prevailing thoughts and knowledge about health and disease);
- staff (including medical, nursing, non-clinical, support, administrative and ancillary);
- finance (both capital for space, buildings and equipment, and revenue for running costs such as staff, consumables and utilities).

Clinical leadership and resources

Since the resources available will never be sufficient to meet every conceivable health need, a key function of the clinical leader is to ensure the appropriate allocation of those that are available.

ABC of Clinical Leadership, 1st edition.
Edited by Tim Swanwick and Judy McKimm. © 2011 Blackwell Publishing Ltd.

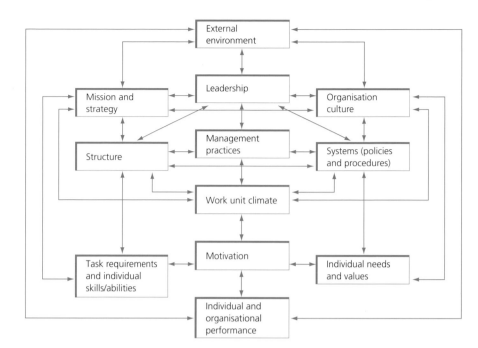

Figure 6.1 Burke-Litwin model of organisational performance and change. *Source*: Burke & Litwin, 1991. Reproduced by permission of W. Warner Burke.

The resource allocation process has two distinct dimensions; at the macro level, governments set policy and decide priorities, with funds distributed by healthcare commissioners; and at the micro level, resources are consumed by individual patients based on multiple decisions of health professionals. Three key criteria apply when allocating clinical resources (Box 6.1).

Box 6.1 **Criteria for allocating clinical resources**

Equity: Ensure that all people who need care have access to services

Allocative efficiency: Ensure that, at both macro and micro levels, funds are not wasted on services which have, relative to other services, low effects on health

Technical efficiency: Ensure that, at the micro level, only the minimum necessary resources are used to deliver a particular activity or set of activities

Source: Black & Gruen, 2005.

Clinical leaders are excellently placed to influence the decisions that health professionals make on a daily basis. They can, for example, ensure that evidence-based medicine is implemented wherever possible, that operating theatre time is allocated optimally and that the best use is made of expensive equipment and facilities over extended hours.

Mission and strategy

Those providing an organisation's vision need to ensure that it is consistent with both its mission and the strategies it has in place to deliver it. Mission, strategy and vision address different organisational questions and operate over different periods (Table 6.1).

Mission focuses on intended outputs and outcomes as well as recognising the inputs required to achieve the outcomes. Strategy

Table 6.1 Mission, strategy and vision.

Concept	Question addressed	Timeframe
Mission	Why does this organisation exist?	Refers to the present. A mission statement provides a brief account of the organisation's purpose
Strategy	How will this organisation deliver its mission?	Usually looks ahead over the next three to five years
Vision	Where does this organisation see itself in the future?	Focuses on a more distant future, gives an indication of where the organisation would like to be and usually presents a substantial challenge

Source: Coghlan & McAuliffe, 2003.

thus provides the link between where we are now (mission) and where we want to be in the future (vision).

The challenge for the clinical leader is not only to spell out the vision but also to ensure that appropriate strategies are developed and implemented.

Organisational culture

There are many definitions of organisational culture. It is sometimes described as 'how things are done around here' or as 'the social and normative glue that holds an organisation together'. Alternatively, culture is 'a set of meanings, ideas and symbols that are shared by members of a collective and have evolved over time'.

Scott *et al.* (2003) point out that the NHS contains many different sub-cultures, and that their relationship to each other and to overall organisational culture is complex (Box 6.2).

Thus managers, physicians, nurses, therapists, clerks, porters, cleaners and other occupational groups each have a distinct sense of identity and purpose. The same is true of other sub-cultures.

Schein (1985) describes three levels of organisational culture, from readily observable artefacts to more intangible assumptions (Figure 6.2). Many attempts have been made to measure culture, and a large number of assessment tools have been developed for use in healthcare organisations. Chapters 12 and 13 discuss gender and culture in more depth.

Clinical leadership and culture

The impact of leadership on organisational culture is central to effective performance. Clinical leaders need to understand the nature of their organisation's culture, know how to assess it and recognise when change is necessary. Key features of culture have been described by Scott *et al.* (2003) (Box 6.3).

Structure

Organisational structure refers to 'the formal division of work and labour, and the formal pattern of relationships that coordinate and control organisational activities' (Bratton, 2007). Structure is most commonly displayed in the form of an organisational chart.

Structure encompasses a number of discrete aspects of organisations, including complexity, formalisation and centralisation (Box 6.4).

Clinical leadership and structure

An understanding of organisational structure is important for clinical leaders as its consequences are far-reaching. Over-specialisation may lead to inefficiency, whilst too little formalisation may mean that essential tasks are not undertaken rigorously enough; and the degree of centralisation has a major impact on levels of motivation, job satisfaction and working relationships.

Substantial research evidence is now available concerning service delivery and organisational issues in healthcare. This has been commissioned by the NIHR Service Delivery and Organisation Research Programme and other bodies. For example, Sheaff *et al.* (2004) reviewed evidence on the impact that organisational arrangements have on the achievement of high performance (Box 6.5).

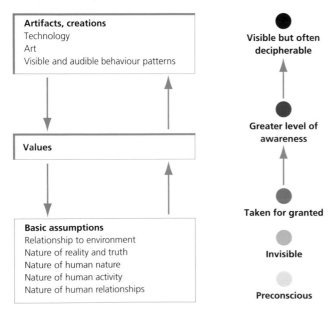

Figure 6.2 Schein's three levels of culture. *Source:* Schein, 1985. Reprinted with permission of John Wiley & Sons, Inc.

Box 6.5 **Clinical leadership and organisational structure**

- **Highly centralized** and bureaucratic organizational structures are not associated with high performance, especially in rapidly-changing settings.
- **Organizational change** needs to be developed from within, not just imposed from outside. Professional engagement and leadership are crucial.
- **Frequent reforms** have made the NHS unstable, leading to falls in performance in some areas of activity.
- **Mergers** may not achieve what matters, such as concentrating expertise or removing duplication.
- **Occupational 'silos'** promote technical change and innovation, but make change management harder.
- The public are reluctant to use **'choice'** to influence the services their GPs provide.
- Governments should be cautious about promoting the use of **for-profit hospitals**.
- **No one-size-fits-all:** local flexibility in organizational arrangements is important to ensure the best fit to local contexts and cultures, which is what improves performance.

Source: Reproduced by permission of the NIHR Service Delivery Organisation Programme Project ref: 08/1318/055. © Queen's Printer and Controller of HMSO 2006.

Management practices

Leadership in healthcare organisations demands an understanding of the running of departments, units or practices; of how managers behave on a day-to-day basis in the delivery of organisational goals; and of the factors that influence that behaviour. These range from the effects of incentives and current management fads to power relations and dynamics in the workplace.

Millward and Bryan (2005) suggest that the practicalities of clinical leadership are best understood in terms of relationships. This means managing the relationships between

- different groups of healthcare professionals;
- healthcare professionals and service users;
- healthcare professionals and the organisations to which they are accountable.

The clinical leader thus needs to have a thorough understanding of the nature of the power relations between the different groups and the dynamics of the relationships between them.

Clinical leadership and power

Clinical leaders have power, authority and influence. To exercise these effectively they need to understand the differences between them and the nature and source of each.

- **Power** concerns the extent to which one individual has influence over another within a certain social system. A has power over B to the extent that they can get B to do something that B would not otherwise do.

Table 6.2 Clinical leadership and power.

Type of power	The extent to which a clinical leader:
Reward	Can use extrinsic and intrinsic rewards to control other people
Coercive	Can deny desired rewards or administer punishment to control other people
Legitimate	Can use the internalised belief of an employee that the 'boss' has a 'right of command' to control other people
Process	Has control over methods of production and analysis
Information	Has control over information needed by others
Expert	Has the ability to control another's behaviour through the possession of knowledge, experience or judgement that the other person needs but does not have

Source: French *et al.*, 2008.

- **Authority** is the power granted by some form of either active or passive consent, whether linked to specific individuals, groups or institutions, which bestows legitimacy on the holder.
- **Influence** encompasses both power and authority, but also embraces effects that are unintended by the clinical leader.

Several types of power exist in organisations, and clinical leaders will have these to varying degrees (Table 6.2).

Leaders need to know under what circumstances to exercise which form of influence or power. They should also be aware of the different kinds of power being exercised by others. These may take many forms, such as hierarchical power exercised by consultants over junior staff, and status power exercised by different medical and surgical sub-specialties, or between doctors and other health professionals.

The relationship between power, authority and influence can be illustrated (Figure 6.3).

Clinical leaders may need to manage the tensions that exist between those with different sources of power, such as between doctors and administrators or finance officers. They may also sometimes be unaware of how much influence they have over the behaviour of others.

Systems

These are the policies and procedures that are in place to facilitate the delivery of the organisation's goals. They include systems for allocating resources, patient information systems and human resource management policies such as recruitment, personal development and appraisal.

Their greatest assets are their staff, and to get the best out of them clinical leaders need to invest in them. It is helpful to make a distinction between human capital and social capital (Table 6.3).

In developing their own staff, clinical leaders should be aware of the differences between leader development and leadership development that exist with reference to human and social capital. For example, Alimo-Metcalfe *et al.* (2007) demonstrate the importance of 'the kind of leadership development that goes beyond developing human capital, and addresses the issue of how best to also

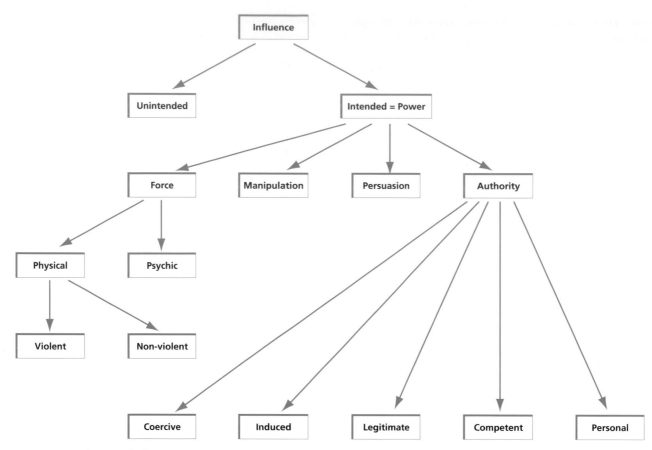

Figure 6.3 Power, authority and influence. *Source*: Bratton, 2007. Reproduced by permission of Palgrave Macmillan, Basingstoke.

Table 6.3 Human and social capital.

Form of capital	Involves	Emphasises
Human capital (individual)	Cognitive skills Emotional skills Self-awareness skills	People are worth investing in as a form of capital; people's performance and the results achieved can be considered as a return on investment
Social capital (group)	Relationships, networking Trust, commitments Appreciation of social and political context	The value of relationships between people, embedded in network links that facilitate trust and communication

Source: Bratton, 2007.

develop social capital, such that leadership becomes embedded in the culture of the team'.

Organisational icebergs

An important role of the clinical leader is to understand how the organisation works as a system, and to ensure that all the parts work in harmony. Effective organisational leadership therefore involves a delicate balancing act in which content issues (policy and evidence-based clinical judgements) have to be juggled with process (clinical delivery) and broader issues such as resource constraints

and service user perspectives. This is a difficult balance to strike, requiring wisdom and judgement as well as knowledge.

If organisations actually worked in the formal, mechanistic way described in organisational charts, life for clinical leaders would doubtless be more straightforward than it is. In reality, organisations lead two lives: the formal public one, as described in organisational charts and procedure manuals, and the informal one, which is

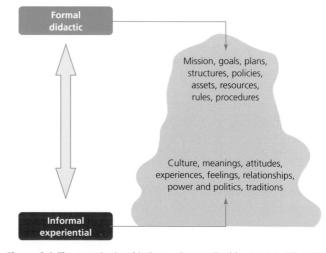

Figure 6.4 The organisational iceberg. *Source*: Coghlan & McAuliffe, 2003. Reproduced by permission of Blackhall Publishing, Blackrock, Ireland.

the lived experience of the organisation. These informal aspects include unofficial working arrangements, social networks at work and battles for influence and authority.

The informal side of an organisation, with its traditions, feelings and attitudes, tends to dominate organisational life, and the phenomenon is sometimes described as the organisational iceberg (Figure 6.4).

Leadership style is the key to getting the best out of individuals. As Alimo-Metcalfe *et al.* (2007) say: 'an engaging style of leadership is what enables the release of human capital, and the creation of social capital'. Leading organisations successfully involves getting the most out of every individual and ensuring that they work effectively together.

References

Alimo-Metcalfe B, Alban-Metcalfe J, Samele C *et al. The Impact of Leadership Factors in Implementing Change in Complex Health and Social Care Environments.* Report to NIHR SDO Programme, SDO/22/2003. 2007.

Black N, Gruen R. *Understanding Health Services.* Open University Press, Maidenhead. 2005.

Bratton J. *Work and Organizational Behaviour.* Palgrave Macmillan, Basingstoke. 2007.

Burke WW, Litwin GH. A causal model of organizational performance and change. *Journal of Management* 1991; **18**(3): 532–45.

Coghlan D, McAuliffe E. *Changing Healthcare Organizations.* Blackhall Publishing, Blackrock, Ireland. 2003.

French R, Rayner C, Rees G, Rumbles S. *Organizational Behaviour.* John Wiley & Sons, Ltd, Chichester. 2008.

Imison C, Giordano RW. Doctors as leaders. *British Medical Journal* 2009; **338**(7701): 979.

Millward LJ, Bryan K. Clinical leadership in health care: A position statement. *Leadership in Health Services* 2005; **18**(2): 13–25.

Schein E. *Organizational Culture and Leadership.* John Wiley & Sons, Inc., London. 1985.

Scott T, Mannion R, Davies H, Marshall M. *Healthcare Performance and Organizational Culture.* Radcliffe Medical Press, Abingdon. 2003.

Sheaff R, Dowling B, Marshall M *et al. Organizational Factors and Performance: A Review of the Literature.* Report to NIHR SDO Programme, SDO/55/2003. 2004.

Further resources

Yukl G. *Leadership in Organizations*, 6th edn. Pearson Prentice Hall, Upper Saddle River, NJ. 2006.

For research reports from the National Institute for Health Research Service Delivery and Organisation Programme see http://www.sdo.nihr.ac.uk/publishedreports.html.

CHAPTER 7

Leading in Complex Environments

David Kernick

St Thomas Medical Group, Exeter, UK

OVERVIEW

- There is no unified science of leadership
- Insights from complexity theory can offer a useful alternative framework when operating in environments of ambiguity and paradox, such as healthcare systems
- Detailed planning and top-down direction of complex systems may prove futile
- In a complex system, emergence is certain but there is no certainty of what will emerge
- The behaviour of complex systems may be profoundly influenced through attention to short-range social processes

Introduction

The way in which we lead is in part determined by our perception of how the system in which we work operates. A useful starting point is to analyse organisations in terms of how well the transfer process (healthcare) that relates inputs (resources) to output (health) is understood, and how well outputs can be defined (Kernick, 2004). See Box 7.1. In the United Kingdom, current policy is to adopt a mixed system, or 'third way', which encourages competition between service providers within a managed healthcare framework. This chapter will consider the implications for leadership if healthcare is viewed as a complex system or 'fourth way'. Here the transfer process is not well understood and the nature of the output of the system – what is health? – is contested.

What is a complex system?

A complex system is a network of elements that exchange information in such a way that change in the context of one element changes the context for all others (Figure 7.1). Negative (damping/stable) and positive (amplifying/unstable) feedback operating re-iteratively give rise to non-linearity. This means that small changes in one area can have large effects across the whole system (the butterfly effect), or conversely large impacts can have little effect. Complex systems cannot be analysed by reducing them into their component parts or

their future predicted or controlled with certainty. This is in contrast with a complicated system, whose action can be determined by an analysis of its component parts and where behaviour is linear and predictable.

Box 7.1 **Four models of health systems**

Inputs (resources) →	Transfer process →	Outputs (health)	Mode of operation
Well understood	Easily measured		Hierarchical, or bureaucratic system: imposed rules and regulations
Poorly understood	Easily measured		Market system: competition, the purchaser/provider split
Partially understood	Partially measured		Mixed system: attempting to get the best of both worlds. Competition within a regulatory framework.
Poorly understood	Not easily measured		Complex adaptive system: 'The Fourth Way'

Source: Kernick, 2004. Reproduced by permission of Radcliffe Medical Press.

Viewing the health service as a complex system and not as a market or bureaucracy can be supported by the fact that

- The nature of the final product, health, is contested.
- There is an often a tenuous relationship between healthcare and health.
- Consumers of healthcare have imperfect knowledge about the product that they receive.
- Managers have an imperfect knowledge of the system they oversee.
- There are unique features of the relationship between the healthcare professional and the patient that include trust and empathy.

ABC of Clinical Leadership, 1st edition.
Edited by Tim Swanwick and Judy McKimm. © 2011 Blackwell Publishing Ltd.

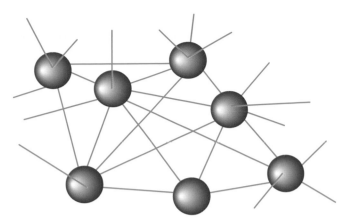

Figure 7.1 Complex system of interacting elements. Changes in one element change the context for all the others.

There are a number of theoretical approaches to complex systems depending on their context and configuration. Human organisations are often viewed as 'complex adaptive systems' – the processing of information by elements changes with time as they learn and adapt in response to other elements or their environment. Some important features of complex systems are shown in Box 7.2 and some implications for a shift to a complexity perspective in organisations shown in Table 7.1.

Box 7.2 **Some important features of complex systems**

- Complex systems consist of a large number of elements that interact. The richness of network connections means that communications will pass across the system but will be modified on the way.
- There are reiterative feedback loops in network interactions giving rise to non-linear features that make the future behaviour of such systems unpredictable.
- It is difficult to determine the boundaries of a complex system. The boundary is often related to the observer's needs and prejudices rather than any intrinsic property of the system itself.
- History is important in complex systems and can determine future behaviour.
- The system is different from the sum of the parts. In attempting to understand a system by reducing it into its component parts, the analytical method destroys what it seeks to understand.
- The behaviour of complex systems evolves from the interaction of agents at a local level without external direction or the presence of internal control. This property is known as emergence and gives systems the flexibility to adapt and self-organise in response to external challenge. Emergence is a pattern of system behaviour that could not have been predicted by an analysis of the component parts of that system.

How can a 'complexity' perspective help clinical leaders?

As discussed in an earlier chapter, leadership is a process of social influence. With complex systems, forms of influence range across a

Table 7.1 Traditional and complexity organisational perspectives.

Traditional organisational perspective	Complexity organisational perspective
Decision made by logical, analytical processes with emphasis on managers controlling and driving strategy. The generation of new ideas is undertaken by experts	Decisions made by exploratory and experimental processes. Intuition and reasoning by analogy encouraged. New ideas can emerge from anyone
Focus on experts and charismatic leaders	Focus on the group. The focus is on the creation of favourable conditions for learning
Importance of future, goal-setting and strategic plans. The focus is on the replication of processes that have worked well elsewhere.	Emphasis is on the here and now. Local structures, processes and patterns are important.
Organisation understood by analysis on component parts	Holistic perspective. The organisation is different from the sum of its parts
Emphasis is on measurement and system quantification	Qualitative aspects of measurement important. The importance of process factors are emphasised as part of a learning process
Attempt to rationalise decision-making even when problems are 'messy', reducing uncertainty and ambiguity	Recognising the creative potential of ambiguity and the importance of resolution through dialogue
Teams are permanent and part of a hierarchical reporting structure. Managers decide who participates and what the boundaries are	Teams are informal, spontaneous and temporary. Participants decide who takes part and what the bounds of their activities are. The focus is on self-organising networks with an appreciation of the importance of both cooperation and competition
Organisation based on strong shared culture	Organisation is provoked and constrained by culture

Source: Kernick, 2004. Reproduced by permission of Radcliffe Medical Press.

spectrum related to the perceived ability of leaders to stand outside of the system and manipulate it towards a pre-defined objective. See Box 7.3.

- *Hard system thinking* is the dominant voice in organisational theory. Here the discourse is of design, regularity and control within the context of a predictable future. Managers stand outside the system and engineer it towards a desired objective, searching for causal links that promise tools for manipulating behaviour. Feedback is used to keep the system from drifting off course, underpinned by mathematical models of the system wherever possible. Leadership is transactional: followers are rewarded (or punished) for their efforts.
- *Soft system thinking* appreciates the differences between the real and modelled world. It is essentially a learning process facilitated by leaders that seeks to converge and reconcile conflicting views of participants in order to derive actions which seem sensible to those concerned but within a framework of stated objectives. Leadership may be transactional or transformational – followers are motivated and mobilised towards a vision.
- *Complexity engineering* sees the leader merging systems theory and complexity insights to manipulate the system in a required direction. The focus is on identifying and changing the simple rules, modulating system attractors or identifying organisational

tipping points where a small input can change the trajectory of the system. Success lies in the ability to recognise and utilise complex and subtle structures amid the wealth of details. Leadership is transformational.

- *Complex responsive processes* approaches are united by a focus on local interaction and the unpredictability of the future. Here the emphasis is on the essentially responsive and participative nature of the human processes of relating and the radical unpredictability of its evolution as we interact with each other in the co-evolution of a jointly constructed reality. The focus is on the 'going on together'. What an organisation is emerges as a result of communication between individuals at a local level. We are always participants in an organisation and can never step outside it to shape it. Leadership is distributed: emergent and without boundaries.

Box 7.3 Case study: Leading change in a complex system

A Director of Quality within a large teaching hospital wants to encourage the participation of medical trainees in quality and safety improvement. He recognises that there are multiple stakeholders and is aware of a number of tensions and drivers within the system, including demands on training time, financial cuts and a drive towards 'metrics-driven' improvement. Despite reluctance from his medical colleagues he includes other healthcare professionals and arranges a series of meetings for colleagues offering only a broad outline of his vision and encouraging discussing how they would approach the issue. He supports and encourages departmental initiatives that emerge even though at times they seem to be at odds with each other. He also facilitates interaction between those involved particularly across professions, inviting expert external input to support promising ideas and challenge the status quo. He sets up a space on the hospital intranet to enable the sharing of good practice and promotes the use of a common set of terms and language. He is supportive when a couple of junior trainees start a hospital newsletter and suggest a series of prizes and awards for projects and departments that he instigates. Things don't seem to be moving forward at the end of the first year until a serious safety issue cuts across a number of departments. This seems to galvanise the hospital and after two years, the project has taken on a life of its own.

What does this mean in practice?

Zimmerman *et al.* (1998) suggest a number of principles developed from a complexity perspective for leaders in healthcare systems.

- **Develop a 'good enough' vision.** Build a good enough vision of the future rather than plan out every little detail. In a non-linear system the future is, in practice, unpredictable and detailed planning is futile.
- **Tune the system to the 'edge of chaos'.** Foster the right degree of information flow, diversity and difference, connections inside and outside the organisation, power differential and anxiety. Uncover and work with paradoxes rather than shying away from them as if they were unnatural. Encourage both cooperation and competition. Let innovation emerge from a creative balanced tension as the system adapts to the configuration that is best suited for the constraints placed upon it.

- **Grow complex systems by 'chunking'.** Allow them to emerge out of links amongst simple systems that work well and are capable of operating independently.
- **Listen to the organisational shadow side.** Informal relationships, gossip and rumour contribute significantly to actions. It is in the shadow system that the 'simple rules' of the system are articulated.
- **Work with 'simple rules'.** This concept is perhaps the most widely used application of complexity insights. The contention is that organisational characteristics emerge from the recursive application of simple rules or guiding principles at a local level (more specifically 'rules of thumb' rather than rules that must be adhered to). Here, the key questions for the leader are: what are the existing and often implicit rules that underpin the existing system; how can they be identified and modified; how can new simple rules be disseminated and introduced? Three types of simple rules for human systems have been proposed: general direction pointing; system prohibition, i.e. setting boundaries; and resource or permission providing. To be accepted, simple rules must have a clear advantage compared with current ways of doing things, be compatible with current system and values, easy to implement and test before making full commitment and the change and its impact must be observable. An example where detailed system specification was replaced by simple rules is shown in Box 7.4.

Box 7.4 Case study: Some simple rules for thrombolysis where a heart attack is suspected and their classification

- Ensure patient receives thrombolysis within sixty minutes of chest pain (*direction pointing*)
- Administration can occur in any environment by a properly trained individual (*direction pointing, boundary setting*)
- Remain within the overall project budget (*boundary setting*)
- Emergency departments and ambulance authorities can draw funding from a pooled budget that has been established to support this change in practice (*resource providing*)

Source: Adapted from Plsek & Wilson, 2001.

Conclusion

A unified science of leadership has proved elusive and its study has merely generated more contested models and theories that remain largely inaccessible to those who actually get on and do the work. The versatile leader will use both linear and non-linear approaches, depending on the context of the task at hand but, ultimately, complexity theory alerts us to the fact that there are no quick policy fixes or any easy way to integrate analytical techniques to leadership processes.

Complexity insights can offer the leader a useful alternative framework when operating in environments of ambiguity and paradox where the focus is on patterns of relationships within organisations, how they are sustained, how they self-organise and how outcomes emerge. If it only sensitises us to the interplay of patterns that perpetually transforms healthcare organisations, it can ameliorate the anxiety of being in command but not in control and help us muddle on together with a little more confidence.

References

Kernick D. An introduction to complexity. In D Kernick (ed.), *Complexity and Health Care Organisation: A View from the Street*. Radcliffe Medical Press, Abingdon. 2004.

Plsek P, Wilson T. Complexity leadership and management in healthcare organisations. *British Medical Journal* 2001; **323**(7315): 746–9.

Zimmerman B, Lindberg C, Plsek P. *Edgeware: Insights from Complexity Science for Healthcare Leaders*. VHA Publishing, Irving, TX. 1998.

Further resources

Axelrod R, Cohen M. *Harnessing Complexity: Organisational implications of a scientific frontier*. Basic Books, New York. 2000.

Griffin R, Stacey R (eds) *Complexity and the Experience of Leading in Organisations*. Routledge/Taylor & Francis, London. 2005.

Lewin R. *Complexity: Life at the Edge of Chaos*. Phoenix, London. 2001.

CHAPTER 8

Leading and Improving Clinical Services

Fiona Moss

NHS London, London, UK

OVERVIEW

- Clinical leadership can profoundly affect the quality of patient care
- Leaders of improvement need a system-wide perspective
- The clinical team is at the heart of quality improvement
- Establishing an organisational culture of continual improvement is crucial to success
- Leaders of improvement need to understand and use quality metrics
- Quality improvement requires healthcare professionals and managers to work collaboratively
- Clinical leaders must have the courage to challenge the status quo and set ambitious goals

---

Introduction

Understanding the relationship between the patient experience, clinical outcomes and the organisation of care is the key to effective clinical leadership. For doctors and nurses trained in the care of individual patients, becoming a leader in the clinical environment requires the translation of a concern for individuals into an appreciation of how the whole system of care contributes to the well-being and care of patients. Professional autonomy and clinical freedom are highly valued by clinicians, but the real benefits of these aspects of clinical practice must be balanced against the benefits of being cared for within an effective organisation. Clinical leaders have a role in defining what professionalism means in an organisational context: managing dedicated clinicians and ensuring the alignment of purpose between managers and healthcare professionals so that care is safe, effective and patient-centred.

Leading for improvement

Much has been written about quality and safety improvement and there are many published examples of successes and sustained improvements. Generating step changes in improvements across the system of care requires a combination of clinical knowledge and understanding coupled with organisational authority and a

ABC of Clinical Leadership, 1st edition.
Edited by Tim Swanwick and Judy McKimm. © 2011 Blackwell Publishing Ltd.

range of organisational skills. The clinical leader is well placed to be at the centre of quality improvement. Indeed, it could be argued that improving the quality and the safety of care should be the clinical leader's main objective and metrics of quality and safety improvement should contribute to the performance indicators of clinical leadership.

Many patients receive healthcare that is appropriate, effective and safe delivered in a timely, patient-centred manner. Research shows, however, that such high-quality care is not delivered consistently and that poor-quality care remains a concern in all healthcare systems. This includes, for example, under-use of effective interventions or use of inappropriate treatments or patients experiencing care that is impersonal. Furthermore, we know that healthcare is endemically *unsafe* with around 14% of patients harmed by the system that sets out to help and heal them. In the United Kingdom, until 1991 when medical audit was introduced, the delivery of good-quality care was an assumed responsibility of individuals and not of the system as a whole. *Medical audit*, which focused on doctors, quickly developed into *clinical audit* as recognition that improvements in care need the input of the whole clinical team. The more recent introduction of *clinical governance* is an acknowledgement of a 'whole system' responsibility for the quality and safety of care and, by implication, for improvements in care. Quality is clearly now a responsibility shared by clinicians and managers, and it falls to the clinical leader to ensure that the objectives of both groups of professionals are aligned and that their efforts are synergistic.

The quality of leadership will profoundly affect the quality of patient care (Berwick, 1989). Good leaders enable the whole organisation to be adaptive and respond to changes from without and within. The changes to the organisation of care necessary for significant and sustained improvements in the quality and safety of care are often complex and time-consuming. The time that it takes to embed organisational change often frustrates clinicians who, even when caring for people with chronic disease, are used to shorter timescales. Effective clinical leaders will seek to sustain clinical colleagues through the ups and downs of the organisational changes that are needed for improvement.

Setting the culture and establishing goals

Broadly, there are two approaches to quality and safety improvement: one that sets out to develop a culture of continuous improvement (Firth-Cozens & Mowbray, 2001) and another centred on a portfolio of top-down projects. Probably both approaches are needed. Establishing a culture in which staff continually seek improvement is a complex but crucial leadership task, one that can only be met if there is a clearly articulated vision and the establishment of a system of organisational values that nurtures and supports individuals, but is intolerant of systemic mistakes. Clinical leaders must work closely with colleagues in human resources to work through, often long-established, cultural barriers to change and to develop an environment in which seeking improvement and expecting demonstrable and sustainable improvements is perceived by all as 'what we do around here'.

Inevitably, leaders will also have to respond to externally imposed imperatives as well as to local priorities, for example waiting list targets set centrally or a local need to reduce length of stay or to improve patient information or to improve access to diabetic service. Good leadership in this context will ensure that teams understand why targets have been set, work together to make the changes and do not simply 'hit the target but miss the point'.

Team working: the heart of quality improvement

The individual clinician-patient relationship is at the heart of healthcare provision. But, as described in Chapter 4, at the heart of quality improvement is the *team*. Teams that work well and whose members experience low stress levels deliver better quality care than poorly functioning teams. Ensuring good team working is an essential task for clinical leaders. In the complex environment of healthcare this may not be straightforward. Some teams are 'real', but many are virtual. For example, routine secondary care investigation of a patient found to have a shadow on a chest radiograph may touch the work of over 20 people, some of whom may not know each other; some will not have seen the patient and yet all must work well together to provide high-quality safe care for this and other patients.

Managing people and supporting the development of the workforce are responsibilities of clinical leaders. Performance management frameworks that link an individual's goals to those of the organisation are potentially useful tools for supporting staff development but may be difficult to use in circumstances where individual staff members belong to several different teams. Furthermore, line management may follow professional hierarchies more closely than it does organisational ones. Continuing and personal development for some staff, in particular doctors and other clinical professionals, may be linked to their speciality and to outside bodies rather than to the immediate needs of the organisation. Such ambiguities that can arise from professionals' different sets of loyalties and identities may have benefits to the organisation, but need to be recognised and acknowledged – and managed. Understanding and resolving such conflicts are some of the tougher challenges of clinical leadership.

Skills needed for quality improvement

Leading clinical improvement requires a set of skills that include skills for leading and managing teams, the ability to understand

work as a series of interdependencies and to lead change across internal and external boundaries (Berwick *et al.*, 1992). Leadership in healthcare systems is distributed, that is within the complexity of healthcare there are many teams and so some individuals will have leadership roles in some but not all aspects of their work. So, the skills needed for quality improvement (Box 8.1) are required by many. Ensuring that everyone understands the nature of improvement and has the necessary skill set should be part of performance management and fall within the remit of the clinical leader.

Box 8.1 **Skills needed for quality improvement**

- Ability to perceive and work in interdependencies
- Ability to work in teams
- Ability to understand work as a process
- Skills in collection, aggregation and analysis of outcome data
- Skills in 'designing' healthcare practices
- Skills in collaborative exchange with patients and with lay managers

Source: Berwick *et al.*, 1992.

Leading improvement requires courage both to challenge the status quo and to set ambitious aims. Such 'stretch goals' serve to highlight the inadequacies of the current system and the need for improvement. But courage is also needed to take those first steps, experiment, initiate pilot projects and set up small plan–do–study–act (PDSA) cycles (Figure 8.1; Langley *et al.*, 1992). Too often, the well-intentioned leader of improvement is overawed by the magnitude of the whole task and distracted by calls for more 'scoping' work, or data collection. In leading improvement, the best is often the enemy of the good.

Risk management and safety improvement

Work on the prevention of accidents in industry has centred on understanding the role of the organisation, and the system

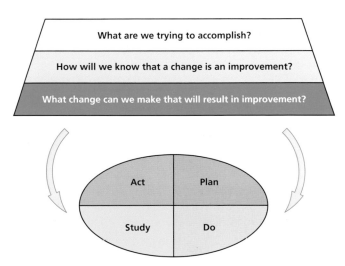

Figure 8.1 A model for improvement. *Source*: Langley *et al.*, 1992.

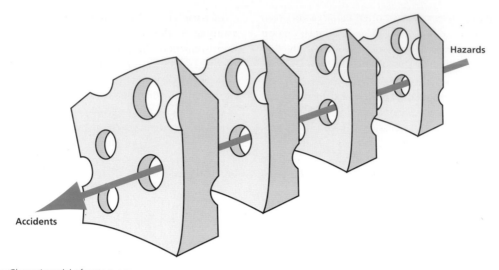

Figure 8.2 The 'Swiss Cheese' model of system error.
The holes in the cheese represent system failures or inadequate defences. When these line up, the result can be catastrophic. *Source*: Reason *et al.*, 2001.

changes needed to make organisations more resilient to accidents and errors. The antecedents of accidents and big failures in health service delivery are usually found to be the product of a series of small errors, each themselves perhaps of little consequence, but when they coincide they produce a massive system failure with the potential for actual harm (Figure 8.2; Reason *et al.*, 2001).

All organisations are, however, the product of the work of individuals. So all individuals should be aware not just of their own role and responsibilities but also of their impact on and contribution to the whole system. In an 'industry' such as health, where the focus is so much on the care and needs of the individual, a task of the clinical leadership for risk management is to train individuals to understand the links between their own individual work and its impact on the system.

In the United Kingdom, after significant failures in the health service there is often an inquiry in order to learn lessons for the future. Analysis of the themes of many inquiries over 30 years (Box 8.2) has identified the factors behind the failures (Walshe & Higgins, 2002).

> ### Box 8.2 **Common themes of inquiries**
>
> - Organisational or geographical isolations: inhibiting transfer of innovation and hindering peer review and constructive critical exchange
> - Inadequate leadership: lacking vision and unwilling to tackle known problems
> - System and process failure: in which organisational systems are either not present or not working properly
> - Poor communication: both within the NHS and between it and patients or clients, which means that problems are not picked up
> - Disempowerment of staff and patients: which means that those that might have raised concerns were discouraged or prevented from doing so
>
> *Source*: Walshe & Higgins, 2002.

Inadequate leadership is one of the top five. Developing good clinical leaders and ensuring they have the skills and the tools to lead multi-professional teams and work with managers so the whole organisation works to shared goals is necessary if patient care is to improve and become safer. Healthcare is likely to be safer if all staff, including junior members of teams, feel enabled to speak out about concerns, acknowledge mistakes and present ideas for improvement. Leaders have a central role in establishing a culture that allows such freedom of expression.

Evidence and measurement

Defining the elements of good-quality care and then measuring these locally is an essential step in quality improvement. Good evidence-based research is essential for the first step and for understanding which interventions should be recommended to patients and is a prerequisite for quality and safety improvement. Simply disseminating the results of clinical research through publication has been found to be relatively ineffective, hence the establishment of the National Institute for Health and Clinical Excellence (NICE), which evaluates and compares the effectiveness of interventions and is now a source of easily accessible guidance and summaries of evidence about interventions.

Measurements of local practice need to be robust enough to be 'owned' and understood by those responsible for care. If local care does not meet best practice, then the results measurements should be used to stimulate discussion about the organisational reasons for the gap between best practice and local care. This can then lead to the formulation of a strategy for change and improvement (Box 8.3). Good clinical leadership is essential in this process to facilitate an understanding of the available 'metrics' and to describe what these mean in relation to the delivery and improvement of care.

Fostering innovation

An important characteristic of healthcare is the continual search for more effective treatments and interventions. But getting research into practice remains a challenge. There is often a long gap between the publication of evidence of the effectiveness of an intervention and its adoption into practice. The 20-year delay in the introduction of thrombolytic therapy, an intervention that significantly reduces mortality from myocardial infarction, is one example. Introducing new interventions usually requires an organisational change. Clinical leaders will need to understand the organisational implications of research findings and facilitate discussion between healthcare professionals and mangers about the costs and benefits of introducing new interventions. It is only when different parts of the organisation are working well together that innovations are likely to be introduced in a timely and effective manner.

Box 8.3 **Case study: Improving repeat prescribing in a general practice**

The staff at a large general practice identified a need to reorganise their repeat prescribing system, which was proving inefficient and frustrating for both staff and patients. An interprofessional quality improvement team was established and a Plan–Do–Study–Act (PDSA) methodology adopted. A target of a 48-hour turnaround time for prescription requests was agreed and the team tested out and implemented a number of measures, including to coincide repeat medications and to record on the computer drugs prescribed during visits, give signing of prescriptions a higher priority and bring them to doctors' desks at an agreed time and move the site for printing prescriptions to the reception desk so as to facilitate face-to-face queries.

Prescription turnaround within 48 hours increased from 95% to 99% at a reduced cost. The number of prescriptions needing records to be looked at was reduced from 18% to 8.6%, saving at least one working day of receptionist time each month. Feedback from all staff indicated greatly increased satisfaction with the newly designed process. The interventions used by the team not only produced measurable and sustainable improvement but also helped the team to learn about the economic costs and benefits and provided them with tools to accomplish their aims.

Source: Cox *et al.*, 1999.

Conclusion

Clinicians know much about the care of patients within their own specialties and are well trained to look after individuals. However, most clinicians receive little formal training in the organisational and leadership skills that may be useful for routine practice but are critical for leading clinical change.

Effective clinical leadership, which requires having an understanding of the whole system of care, is vital for continuous improvement in the quality and the safety of care and for assuring the safe and timely introduction of new interventions. Good clinical leaders unite clinicians and managers and their agendas and are thus key to the development of a healthy organisational structure, fit to deliver effective, safe and patient-centred care. Clinical leaders have a vital place in modern healthcare. They need a wide range of skills if they are to fulfil their roles and inspire, promote, manage and sustain change and improvement in a complex system that involves many people.

References

Berwick D. Continuous quality improvement: An ideal in health care. *New England Journal of Medicine* 1989; **320**: 53–6.

Berwick D, Enthoven A, Bunker JP. Quality management in the NHS: The doctor's role. *British Medical Journal* 1992; **304**(6821): 235–9.

Cox S, Wilcock P, Young J. Improving the repeat prescribing process in a busy general practice: A study using continuous quality improvement methodology. *Quality in Health Care* 1999; **8**: 119–25.

Firth-Cozens J, Mowbray D. Leadership and the quality of care. *Quality in Health Care* 2001; **10**(suppl. 2): ii3–ii7.

Langley GJ, Nolan KM, Nolan TW. *The Foundation of Improvement*. API Publishing, Silver Spring, MD. 1992.

Reason J, Carthey J, de Leval MR. Diagnosing the 'vulnerable system syndrome': An essential pre-requisite to effective risk management. *Quality in Health Care* 2001; **10**(suppl. 2): ii21–ii25.

Walshe K, Higgins J. The use and impact of inquiries in the NHS. *British Medical Journal* 2002; **353**(7369): 895–900.

Further resources

Health Quality Council and National Primary Care Development Team. Quality Improvement Toolbook. 2010, http://www.chsrf.ca/kte_docs/Quality%20Improvement%20Toolbook.pdf, accessed 1 May 2010.

Institute of Healthcare Improvement. How to Improve. 2010, www.ihi.org/IHI/Topics/Improvement/ImprovementMethods/HowToImprove/, accessed 1 May 2010.

NHS Institute for Innovation and Improvement. Quality and Service Improvement Tools for the NHS. 2010, http://www.institute.nhs.uk/quality_and_service_improvement_tools/quality_and_service_improvement_tools/quality_and_service_improvement_tools_for_the_nhs.html, accessed 19 July 2010.

Scottish Government. A Guide to Service Improvement. 2010, www.scotland.gov.uk/Publications/2005/11/04112142/21428, accessed 1 May 2010.

CHAPTER 9

Educational Leadership

Judy McKimm[1] *and Tim Swanwick*[2]

[1]Unitec, Auckland, New Zealand
[2]London Deanery, London, UK

> **OVERVIEW**
>
> - Leadership occurs at all levels in clinical education, from one-to-one supervision through to leading complex educational organisations
> - Clinical education is a 'crowded stage' involving NHS, university and other public service sectors
> - To be effective, educational leaders require a good understanding of health service delivery, higher-education management, quality assurance and funding mechanisms
> - Traditional professional roles and boundaries are being challenged by health service needs
> - Leadership in clinical education is ultimately for the benefit of patients – both today and tomorrow

Introduction

Clinical educators carry the double burden of managing and leading teams and institutions in a rapidly changing educational environment whilst working in close collaboration with a range of healthcare professionals to deliver safe and high-quality patient care. In this chapter we consider the context for healthcare education, and discuss current educational systems and structures and corresponding leadership roles in medical and health professional education. Challenges for educational leaders are discussed, which include leading across boundaries, funding and commissioning, interprofessional education, changing professional roles, the impact of learning technologies, widening participation and diversity.

The education policy context

Clinical education straddles higher education and health services, both arenas of rapid change. Responding to a seemingly never-ending stream of policy and strategic agendas (summarised in Box 9.1) poses huge challenges.

Higher education agendas such as lifelong learning, inclusivity and widening participation have resulted in a larger and more diverse learner population. Technological advances, such as simulation, e-learning and m-learning (mobile learning), have provided impetus for the development of new modes of educational delivery. E-learning and the use of mobile devices offer solutions for managing increased student numbers in diverse geographical and clinical locations. But clinical education is also profoundly affected by health service changes. Workforce planning, funding and commissioning arrangements are increasingly complex, requiring new skills from clinical leaders and managers as they engage with a range of different bodies including 'patient partnerships'. Service reconfiguration and the implementation of integrated services and the devolution of services to local communities, means that 'where' and 'how' learners learn is changing. Different types of health workers are needed and traditional healthcare roles are being challenged.

Crucially, increased student numbers and service changes have resulted in a reduction of learner access to patients and direct clinical experience. Although simulated environments such as clinical and communication skills laboratories provide alternatives, planning and delivering the workplace-based clinical education required by professional bodies and, indeed, patients is increasingly difficult, requiring ever more creative solutions and 'agile curricula'.

> **Box 9.1 Policy drivers for clinical education**
>
> - Increasing student numbers
> - Modularisation of programmes
> - Increased access to flexible education and training
> - Diversity of learner population
> - Technological advances e.g. e-learning, simulation
> - Accountability for educational quality
> - Changing profile of service delivery:
>   - shift to community settings
>   - integrated services
>   - faster throughput with reduced patient access
> - Changing workforce planning, funding and commissioning
> - Professionalisation of clinical education – 'training the trainers'
> - Empowerment of patients – 'patients as partners'
> - Redefinition of professional roles

ABC of Clinical Leadership, 1st edition.
Edited by Tim Swanwick and Judy McKimm. © 2011 Blackwell Publishing Ltd.

Structures in clinical education

Educational leadership is played out across three sectors: undergraduate (or pre-registration), postgraduate (post-registration) and continuing professional development. Although each healthcare profession has its own unique set of educational structures and processes, there are similarities across the disciplines. Broadly speaking, six key functional areas can be identified:

- funding;
- commissioning;
- providing;
- regulating;
- standard setting;
- licensing.

As an example, Box 9.2 outlines the bodies responsible for these functions in medical education in England.

Box 9.2 **Structure and function in medical education in England**

Sector / Function	Undergraduate	Postgraduate	Continuing professional development
Funding	National Health Service and Higher Education Funding Council England	Department of Health and NHS employer	Individual or NHS employer
Commissioning	Higher Education Funding Council England (direct student numbers) Department of Health (indirect, linked to workforce planning)	Strategic Health Authorities via Deaneries	Individual or NHS employer
Providing	Universities (direct) Health and other services (indirectly, via universities)	Deaneries via Specialty and Foundation Schools	Independent providers e.g. Universities, Royal Medical Colleges
Regulating	General Medical Council and Quality Assurance Agency	General Medical Council*	May be regulated by employer or through professional appraisal processes
Standard setting	General Medical Council	General Medical Council* informed by Royal Medical Colleges	General Medical Council Colleges
Licensing and relicensing	N/A	General Medical Council	General Medical Council

*Formerly the responsibility of the Postgraduate Medical Education and Training Board (PMETB).

The formal leadership of healthcare education may be exercised from a number of organisations or agencies, such as professional bodies, colleges, universities, government, the NHS, strategic health authorities and trusts. Increasingly we see collaboration between institutions and authorities developing as a way of achieving 'buy in' to strategic initiatives. The development of the *Medical Leadership Competency Framework* – collaboration between the NHS Institute for Innovation and Improvement and the Academy of Medical Royal Colleges – is a good example (Academy of Medical Royal Colleges/NHS Institute for Innovation and Improvement, 2008).

On the ground, all clinical educators need to be involved in leadership. In practice though, this activity tends to be aligned with particular job roles, such as college or undergraduate tutor, training programme director, associate dean, university lecturer, professor or head of department or school. Increasing numbers of clinicians are trained in teaching and learning but a persisting concern is that leaders in clinical education are often promoted to positions of influence without formal educational qualifications and, more often than not, without any managerial or leadership experience.

Integration of education with service delivery

One of the major challenges for leaders of clinical education is the integration of service and educational delivery. This has always been an essential feature of most health professional education and training but has become more of a challenge in recent years. Not only does work-based learning have considerable educational validity, but it is also essential for preparing students for practice. Increasingly, graduates find themselves unprepared for the real world. This realisation has led to a range of initiatives such as early clinical contact in the undergraduate years, increased patient involvement and a focus on work-based teaching, learning and assessment.

A number of important issues arise. Workplace-based teaching and learning creates strains on services already struggling to cope with a target-driven agenda, patient safety is an increasing concern and there are implications for staffing and resources. Truly integrating education with service relies on clinicians to deliver education, a task that is not their primary role and for which they may be ill prepared. Leaders of clinical education need to understand and work across the education–service interface, and boundaries between organisations, professions, subject disciplines and professions, to influence, enable and set the conditions to make work-based learning possible.

Professional roles and responsibilities: the changing shape of the health workforce

In response to policy shifts and service changes, traditional professional identities are being redefined. In the past, health professions' training was carried out uni-professionally with a relatively clear understanding on what the future role of those professionals might entail. But this situation is changing. Although most undergraduate health professional programmes are still designed to produce, for example, doctors, nurses or pharmacists, programmes aimed at producing new health and social care workers are being introduced, such as mental health practitioners dually qualified and registered as social workers and mental health nurses. The number of health and related 'professions' has correspondingly increased as roles such as paramedic, operating department practitioner and physician's assistant are professionalised through degree-level education and nationally regulated training programmes.

At post-qualification level, two additional changes are occurring as traditional roles and responsibilities of qualified practitioners are extended through the creation of advanced practitioners such as nurse consultants and prescribing pharmacists, alongside an increasingly distributed and team-based approach to patient care. The wider impact of these workforce changes on service, education and the identity and requirements of traditional professions is as yet unclear, but educational leaders need to be vigilant to the tensions posed by the continual reshaping of professional roles and boundaries.

Interprofessional education

Although educational trends come and go, interprofessional education, where learners from different groups 'learn with, from and about one another' (CAIPE, 2006), has been endorsed by the World Health Organization (2010) as underpinning team working and, in turn, improving health outcomes. Interprofessional education reflects the working and communication patterns in real clinical practice and so gives opportunities for learners to practise skills and develop these relationships in a relatively safe environment. However, delivering interprofessional education in a busy service context where learners still tend to be taught by members of their own profession is challenging (Freeth, 2008). Box 9.3 summarises the advantages of interprofessional education and barriers to its delivery and Box 9.4 describes how some of these barriers can be overcome.

Box 9.3 **Interprofessional education: advantages and barriers**

Advantages	Barriers
• Encourages learners to learn about different health care roles and responsibilities	• Logistics can be difficult with competing timetables and clinical placements
• Develops respect for other professional attributes and roles	• Uni-professional training programmes tend to maintain working in professional 'silos'
• Develops professional identity in relation to other health professionals	• Needs good facilitation from a range of different health professionals
• Develops skills in team working and collaboration	• Can lead to increased stereotyping if not well facilitated
• Improves patient care	• Some students (and teachers) do not see the benefit
• Improves health outcomes	

Box 9.4 **Case study: Leading interprofessional education**

A health sciences faculty in a large university has three separate programmes for medical, nursing and pharmacy students. The Dean of Education wishes to introduce interprofessional education because she feels that students would be advantaged in learning to work with, and from, other health professional students at an early stage. After reading the literature and considering the barriers and constraints, she decides to involve key stakeholders from all departments, and students, in a group to plan how interprofessional education might be introduced. After some considerable negotiation, the group is persuaded to introduce a brand new initiative for all health professional students in the first week of their study at the university. The 'freshers week' initiative includes formal education, social events and an introduction to studying at the university. The initiative is very successful and paves the way for further events linked to common learning outcomes which run throughout the curricula of all three programmes.

Accountability vs. autonomy

The teacher, like the artist, the philosopher and the man of letters, can only perform his work adequately if he feels himself to be an individual directed by an inner creative impulse, not dominated and fettered by an outside authority. (Russell, 2009)

Bertrand Russell's observation encapsulates a key dilemma for the leader of clinical education who has to tread a fine line between *accountability* and *autonomy*: working responsively but creatively with policy, monitoring and maintaining standards, whilst allowing clinical teachers the freedom they need to innovate and work imaginatively with learners. In fact, this balancing act is systemic throughout higher and professional education as curricula and standards have become increasingly centralised and responsibility for interpretation and delivery pushed out to the periphery. Examples of centrally determined and developed curricula or frameworks which require providers of education with an obligation for delivery include the General Medical Council's (2009) recommendations on undergraduate medical education, *Tomorrow's Doctors*, and the Postgraduate Medical Education and Training Board's (2008) standards for clinical and educational supervisors.

Resource management

A key activity and challenge for clinical leaders is identifying and managing the human and physical resources required to deliver education when learning opportunities with patients are increasingly restricted. In clinical education, funding comes from a range of sources within and external to the organisation, department or service. Leaders need to be aware of the opportunities that exist for providing effective ('it works') and efficient ('within budget') clinical education. The complexity of resource

	Option 1 'do nothing'	Option 2	Option 3
Advantages/benefits			
Disadvantages/costs			
Net effects			
Risks			

Figure 9.1 Options appraisal.
This tool, used in conjunction with a risk matrix, enables you to quantify and agree the impact and the risks of each of the options available. Remember to always include 'do nothing' as one of the options.

management should not be underestimated, particularly when the clinical setting includes learners from different professional groups and at different levels, all of whom may well be funded from different sources. Problems of educational delivery can usually be solved by collaboration, imagination, willingness to work in different ways and understanding both of where funding may be obtained and how educational methods (such as e-learning) can be used creatively and flexibly. Involving different professional groups, sponsors or collaborating with other organisations can optimise the development and utilisation of major teaching facilities such as skills centres or simulation suites. Decisions involving major investment need to be appraised in terms of long-term sustainability, potential risk and options (Figures 9.1 and 9.2). Leaders often find that

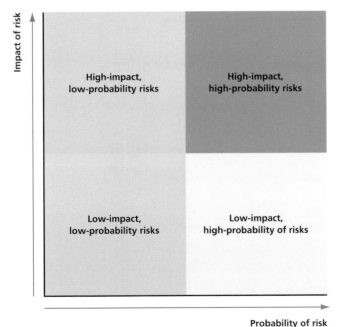

Figure 9.2 The risk matrix.
Assess risks according their impact and their probability. Balance risks so that few (if any) activities fall into the top right square and that most activities fall into the bottom left square.

decisions have to be 'satisfied' (agreed within constraints) and accept that the result is often a compromise.

Leading professional colleagues

Leading professional colleagues is never easy – 'herding cats' is a commonly deployed description – and professional organisations themselves tend to be sluggish to respond to change. In Henry Mintzberg's (1992) comparative anatomy of organisations, *Structure in Fives*, he points out that changes in the behaviour of professionals within the organisation's 'operating core' result from a slow and gradual shift in norms and values brought about by interactions between members, or more usually by new blood coming into the organisation (Figure 9.3). Unlike other organisational forms such as those found in industrial or commercial companies, the standards for professionals are normally set outside the organisation by, for instance, medical colleges or professional associations, and professionals work to these standards exercising a high degree of autonomy. As a result, strategy in a professional organisation tends to represent an accumulation of projects or initiatives that individual members are able to convince it to undertake. The message here for those that attempt to lead change and improvement in clinical education is that 'command and control' is an ineffective leadership style and top-down plans and diktats rarely result in lasting and deep-rooted change.

Challenges for leaders of clinical education

A summary of some of the key challenges identified for leaders of clinical education is presented in Box 9.5 (McKimm, 2004). Being aware of these challenges and seeking ways to address them at individual, team and organisational levels will provide leaders of education with a checklist and framework for action. The students of today are the practitioners of tomorrow, and so there is a professional obligation on all clinicians to be involved with teaching, supervision and training activities. The current emphasis on embedding leadership at all levels emphasises the need for everyone to take some sort of educational leadership role. Despite the

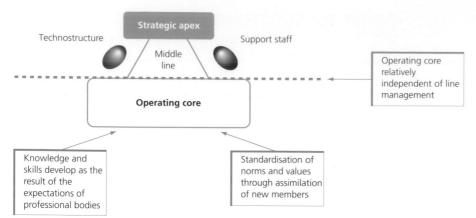

Figure 9.3 The professional organisation. *Source*: Mintzberg, 1992.

challenges, leading clinical education activities and initiatives (at whatever level) is not only a core component of professional life but can often be one of the most rewarding. Support is provided to extend teaching knowledge and skills from universities, postgraduate centres and postgraduate deaneries, which can also assist health service leaders in gaining an understanding of the principles and practice of clinical education. Coupled with a wider awareness of education structures and management systems, an understanding of leadership and management roles and a willingness to collaborate to meet learners' needs should result in the provision of high-quality learning opportunities, delivered in accordance with the needs of health services, students and peers.

Box 9.5 Challenges for leaders of clinical education

Personal issues

- Maintaining an appropriate work life balance
- Culture of senior management practice impacts on career progression for those with domestic responsibilities
- For women:
  - issues concerning career breaks
  - domestic commitments
  - the 'glass ceiling'
- Difficult to manage clinical and senior educational commitments
- Decisions over leaving clinical practice are tied in with maintaining credibility as a leader
- Educational role often undervalued by organisations

Organisational and cultural issues

- Need to understand the history and anthropology of their own organisation, organisational strengths and function
- Managing and leading people, ensuring they are in the right roles and positions
- Work life balance issues, culture and work ethos
- Hierarchical and centrally controlled structures can impede change management
- Some clinicians find it difficult to reduce clinical workloads and make the shift into educational roles

Balancing competing agendas

- Overwhelming issue is working with the rapid and complex changes affecting the NHS: difficult to make long term decisions or contracts
- Dual demands of working in HE, which is very accountable, and an NHS undergoing rapid change puts greater strain on health care education leaders than in other sectors of HE
- Conflict between the core values and demands of the NHS (patient led, service driven) and those of HE (student and research led)
- Management styles differ between universities and the NHS. University staff can resent over-management and seek autonomy, whereas NHS staff are more used to working in formal hierarchies with vertical management styles
- A 'crowded stage' with multiple task masters: leaders have to predict and meet the needs of the NHS and HE, enabling staff to deal with universities and the NHS through partnership and collaboration
- Healthcare education leaders have to deal with the needs of professional and statutory, quality assurance and funding bodies
- Difficult to motivate clinicians with heavy clinical workloads, and academics who are being pushed into generating research output

The wider agenda

- Healthcare education leaders have an influential role in changing and improving healthcare systems and structures through partnership and education
- Awareness of wider educational agendas helps leaders to drive and address issues such as interprofessional learning, diversity and promoting innovation in learning strategies

Source: McKimm 2004.

References

Academy of Medical Royal Colleges/NHS Institute for Innovation and Improvement. *Medical Leadership Competency Framework*. NHS Institute of Innovation and Improvement, London. 2008.

CAIPE (UK Centre for the Advancement of Interprofessional Education). CAIPE reissues its statement of the definition and principles of interprofessional education. *CAIPE Bulletin* 2006; **26**: 3, http://www.caipe.org.uk/about-us/defining-ipe/, accessed 13 July 2010.

Freeth D. Interprofessional education. In: T Swanwick (ed.), *Understanding Medical Education*. Wiley-Blackwell, Chichester. 2010.

General Medical Council. *Tomorrow's Doctors*. GMC, London. 2009.

McKimm J. *Case Studies in Leadership in Medical and Health Care Education: Special Report 5*. Higher Education Academy Subject Centre for Medicine, Dentistry and Veterinary Medicine, Newcastle-upon-Tyne. 2004.

Mintzberg H. *Structure in Fives: Designing effective organisations*. Prentice Hall, Harlow. 1992.

Postgraduate Medical Education and Training Board. *Educating Tomorrow's Doctors: Future models of medical training: Medical Workforce Shape and Trainee Expectations*. PMETB, London. 2008.

Russell B. *Unpopular Essays*. Routledge, London. 2009.

World Health Organization. *Framework for Action on Interprofessional Education and Collaborative Practice*. WHO, Geneva. 2010.

Further resources

Bush T. *Theories of Educational Leadership and Management*, 3rd edn. Sage, London. 2003.

Darzi A. *A High Quality Workforce: NHS Next Stage Review*. Department of Health, London. 2008.

Department of Health. *High Quality Care for All: The NHS Next Stage Review Final Report*. The Stationery Office, London. 2009.

McKimm J, Swanwick T. Educational leadership. In: T Swanwick (ed.), *Understanding Medical Education*. Wiley-Blackwell, Chichester. 2010.

CHAPTER 10

Leading for Collaboration and Partnership Working

Judy McKimm

Unitec, Auckland, New Zealand

> ### OVERVIEW
>
> - Collaboration and partnership working are related but different concepts
> - Integrated and community-based services require new ways of working and new forms of leadership
> - Collaborative practice and team working improves health outcomes and patient experience
> - Collaborative leadership involves working across organisational, functional, professional and sectoral boundaries to improve patient care
> - Collaborative leadership is an effective strategy for complex situations

Introduction

Collaborative leadership is a key approach in integrated public services with complex funding arrangements and increasing accountability. The moves towards more joined-up working bring opportunities and challenges for clinical leadership, requiring a broad-based understanding of systems, organisations, communities and people, coupled with a willingness to work and lead in new ways.

What is collaboration and partnership?

The terms 'collaboration' and 'partnership' are often used interchangeably, but they are defined differently. Collaboration is a *process* involving 'a philosophical and cultural commitment to the principles and practice of partnership working in the shared interest of better outcomes for the end-user and the whole community' (McKimm *et al.*, 2008). Outcomes are enabled through

- joint decision-making among interdependent parties;
- joint ownership of decisions;
- collective responsibility for outcomes;
- working across professional and functional boundaries;
- establishing supporting factors such as resources, systems and processes (Liedtka & Whitten, 1998).

ABC of Clinical Leadership, 1st edition.
Edited by Tim Swanwick and Judy McKimm. © 2011 Blackwell Publishing Ltd.

Partnership describes the *relationships* that need to be achieved, maintained and reviewed, often through formalised, legal agreements.

The policy context

Participative and collaborative clinical leadership is enshrined in the wider public service policy context. The 'modernisation agenda' (the NHS policy 'supertanker') emphasised greater accountability of professionals and organisations, taking a managerial approach through the reconfiguration of services, the implementation of measures including target setting and 'best value' and the appointment of non-clinical managers. This approach had positive effects in terms of alignment of budgets and the improvement of some health outcomes, but led to disconnect between clinicians and managers and deficits in clinical leadership and governance (Imison & Giordano, 2009).

A series of inquiries emphasising the failure of health systems and professionals to care for society's most vulnerable people set the agendas for integrated, community-based public services in motion, establishing Integrated Children's Services (resulting primarily from the Laming report, Laming, 2003), disability, mental health and adult integrated services. 'New managerialism' was therefore tempered by policy shifts which devolved services to communities and reconfigured traditional professional roles in the light of the skills mix required to deliver new services. *Next Stage Review* (Department of Health, 2009), the 'personalisation agenda' (Department of Health, 2008) and calls for doctors in particular to take back the mantle of clinical leadership (Imison & Giordano, 2009) have set the scene for the reconsideration of clinical leadership and its role in delivering modern health services.

Collaborative practice

Collaborative practice is when multiple health and care workers from different professional backgrounds work together with patients, families, carers and communities to deliver the highest quality comprehensive care services. The World Health Organization (WHO) endorses that collaborative practice improves health outcomes and strengthens health systems (World Health Organization, 2007). A strong, flexible and collaborative workforce is essential to address major health challenges such as ageing populations and management of long-term conditions. The global system shift from individualist to collectivist approaches embeds collaborative leadership in leadership frameworks, working practices and research endeavours. Cross-disciplinary team working, co-creation of knowledge and sharing practice are essential. Box 10.1 describes how the WHO defines interdependent components of complex health systems.

Box 10.1 **The six building blocks of a health system**

Good **health services** are those which deliver effective, safe, quality personal and non-personal health interventions to those that need them, when and where needed, with minimum waste of resources.

A well-performing **health workforce** is one that works in ways that are responsive, fair and efficient to achieve the best health outcomes possible, given available resources and circumstances (i.e. there are sufficient staff, fairly distributed; they are competent, responsive and productive).

A well-functioning **health information** system is one that ensures the production, analysis, dissemination and use of reliable and timely information on health determinants, health system performance and health status.

A well-functioning health system ensures equitable access to essential **medical products, vaccines and technologies** of assured quality, safety, efficacy and cost-effectiveness, and their scientifically sound and cost-effective use.

A good **health financing** system raises adequate funds for health, in ways that ensure people can use needed services, and are protected from financial catastrophe or impoverishment associated with having to pay for them. It provides incentives for providers and users to be efficient.

Leadership and governance involves ensuring strategic policy frameworks exist and are combined with effective oversight, coalition-building, regulation, attention to system-design and accountability.

Source: World Health Organization, 2007.

Benefits of collaboration

The benefits of collaborative practice in acute, primary and community settings are well evidenced, summarised in Box 10.2 (World Health Organization, 2007).

Box 10.2 **Benefits of collaborative practice**

The benefits of collaborative practice include:

- Improved patient care:
  - higher levels of satisfaction
  - better acceptance of care
  - improved health outcomes
- Improved access to and coordination of health services
- More appropriate use of specialist clinical resources and of scare resources (e.g. in rural or remote areas)
- Increase in safety and reduction of clinical errors

- Decrease in:
  - total patient complications
  - length of hospital stay and duration of treatment
  - hospital admissions
  - outpatient and clinic visits
  - mortality rates
  - staff turnover
  - overall cost of care
- Grants and funding are often geared towards collaboration and partnership working, thus supporting non-core service improvements and innovations.

Source: World Health Organization, 2007.

The risks to patient care when health professionals don't (won't or can't) collaborate are immense. Improved health outcomes often depend on health and non-health workers collaborating in achieving broader health determinants such as better housing, clean water, food, security, education and a violence-free society. The recent case in the UK of 'Baby P' – a 17-month old who died after suffering more than 50 injuries over an eight-month period, during which he was repeatedly seen by local childrens' services and health professionals – is just one example of the failure of health and other professionals to collaborate and communicate effectively. Collaborative leaders need to be 'system aware', 'collaborative practice ready' and think outside the confines of health and health systems (World Health Organization, 2007 and 2010).

Leadership approaches

Collaborative leadership sits within the 'new paradigm' approaches which include transformational, situational (or contingent), dispersed or distributed, and value-led leadership (see Chapter 3). In particular, it reflects Greenleaf's (1977) 'servant leadership', in which serving the organisation, profession or sector takes precedence over the urge to lead. Traditional views of leadership are being challenged and, although there is no coherent or consistent

Table 10.1 Traditional and alternative perceptions of leadership.

The traditional view	The alternative view
Leadership resides in individuals	Leadership is a property of social systems
Leadership is hierarchically based, linked to position	Leadership can occur anywhere, 'at all levels'
Leadership occurs when leaders do things to followers	Leadership is a complex process of mutual influence
Leadership is different from and more important than management	The leadership/management distinction is not important
Leaders are different and have certain personal qualities	Anyone can be a leader
Leaders are born	Leadership can be learnt
Leaders make a crucial difference to organisational performance	Leadership is one of many factors that influence organisational performance
Effective leadership is generalisable	The context of leadership is crucial

Source: Adapted from Simkins, 2004.

view on what might replace them, Simkins and others (Simkins, 2004) have identified some of the key shifts (Table 10.1).

Personal skills

Collaborative leaders may need to draw on personal authority and qualities rather than positional power, particularly when working across organisations, sectors or professional boundaries when their organisational role or professional qualification may not be relevant (Box 10.3). Working in interprofessional teams (see Chapter 4) requires different leadership approaches and active followership. Establishing credibility amongst people or groups with very different values and ways of working takes time, effort and emotional labour.

Box 10.3 **Personal skills for collaboration**

- Being able to apologise
- Balancing humility with gaining trust and credibility
- Advocating your point of view without harming your collaborator's feelings
- Being clear, avoiding ambiguity and duplication of effort
- Spotting when a conversation gets emotional and then making it safe again to continue meaningful dialogue
- Active listening and 'walking in the shoes' of your collaborator
- Finding the common ground, asking questions and requesting examples that illustrate what is meant
- Defining a mutual intent that will inspire action
- Telling and eliciting stories, conversation, dialogue and 'polylogue'
- Being able to get things done, so you have something to show for your collaboration ('visible wins')
- Networking, being a 'connector', knowing people and systems
- Showing that you are willing to learn and don't know everything
- Being able to live with outcomes that may not be what you anticipated or wanted as long as they improve patient care or outcomes
- Being resilient

Collaborative leaders also lead by example through demonstrating commitment to the process and outcomes of the collaboration and supporting others in collaborative initiatives, system developments or service improvements.

Culture and change

Culture is 'the way we do things here'. At the organisational or professional level, ensuring that the 'culture' works effectively to support collaboration is a major challenge. Classic views, such as Lewin's 'unfreeze – change – refreeze' model (Lewin, 1951), of change management saw culture as a thing, as a 'state', offering techniques such as organisational development to help leaders (change agents) 'manage' change.

Current concepts, based on social constructivist theory, see culture as constantly mediated: the emergent result of continuing negotiations and conversations about values and meanings. If you want to change cultures towards those that value and promote

collaboration, then systems, processes, conversations and stories need to be changed. Collaborative working appears to occur from deep within systems when the conditions are favourable. This requires open dialogue and 'polylogue' – multiple, tempered, 'fierce conversations' – essential for teasing out and challenging existing work practices (Lee-Davies *et al.*, 2007).

Collaboration is often effective in complex situations where emergent change occurs through 'perturbing the edge of chaos' (see Chapter 7). Snowden and Boone's (2007) model can be used for making management and leadership decisions in different situations (Figure 10.1).

Leading collaboratively to effect change

Collaborative leaders ensure that all people affected by a decision (the stakeholders) are part of the change process. Collaborative initiatives require the early identification of all stakeholders so that opportunity can be provided for input, influence and the exchange of ideas through establishing communication systems and building in time for discussion, responses and change. This is where the 'philosophical commitment' to collaboration is most challenging, especially when there is pressure from funding bodies or more senior managers for quick changes and early completion.

Power, authority and influence

Many people feel that power is somehow a dirty word. Collaborative leaders need to be comfortable with gaining and using power and influence, whilst being alert to potential misuses of power. Partnerships or collaborations usually involve an imbalance of power, relating to financial or other resources; formal leadership of the initiative (bestowed, legitimate power); individual or organisational track record or status (referent power); professional knowledge (expert power) or accountability arrangements (e.g. for funding).

Effective leadership requires credibility to be established, often with individuals and groups with different goals, values or histories. Personal maturity and a new notion of power which does not fear loss of control enables power sharing: the power of a collaboration is stronger than the sum of its parts (Figure 10.2). Kanter (1982) suggests that power can be 'gained through giving' by giving people: important work to do, discretion and autonomy, visibility and recognition and by building relationships.

The leadership 'gap'

Different players in healthcare teams may have very different expectations of leadership roles and behaviours. Medical leadership (in common with other leadership forms in large, hierarchical organisations) has traditionally been 'command and control' leadership. And whilst senior doctors frequently have ultimate clinical responsibility for patients and manage resources, the shift towards more integrated care services led and managed by other (not necessarily health) professionals means that this is increasingly not the case. Adopting traditional leadership approaches may mean that clinicians are out of step with the way in which flatter, interprofessional and collaborative teams need to work (Figure 10.3).

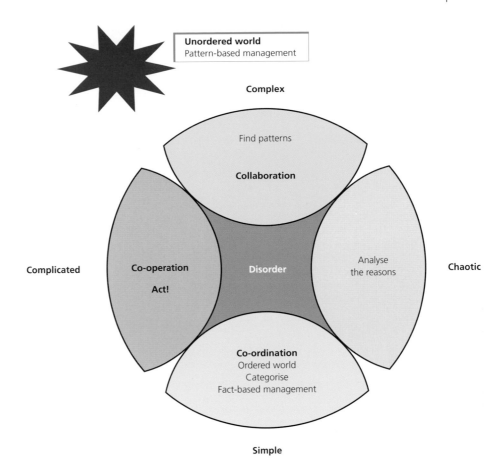

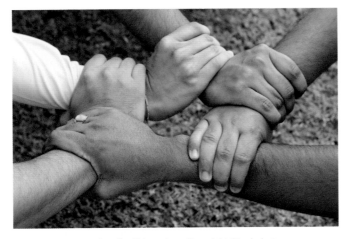

Figure 10.2 Strengths of collaboration. Copyright iStockphotos.

New systems and new ways of working

Truly adept leaders know not only how to identify the context they're working in, but also how to change their behaviour to match. (Snowden & Boone, 2007).

Alongside traditional organisations, new systems have been established that rely less on organisational status and more on relationships formed through informal interdependency:

- Networks and meshworks – loose-coupled people and systems, relying on forming relationships required through 'interactions'

around shared values, visions, ideas and projects. These include managed clinical networks (e.g. in cancer care);
- Alliance – a union of interests that have similar character, structure or outlook;
- Coalition – a temporary alliance of parties for some specific purpose;
- Consortium – association, a group of similar interests;
- Communities of practice – a model of collaborative, situational working where members work towards a common goal defined in terms of knowledge, rather than task (Wenger, 1998).

Research into Integrated Children's Services identifies three types of leadership and management role for effective service delivery: operational (gets things done), coordinator and policy-maker and strategist (thinking role). 'Co-ordination roles [are] about working with others, collaborating, networking, gaining trust and respect, and building effective relationships' (Hartle *et al.*, 2008).

Many of the activities of collaborative leaders occur in the 'spaces between' organisations, professions, departments and functions. New types of leaders are needed who are comfortable working in the spaces and across boundaries, removing barriers to achieve shared vision and dealing with complex 'wicked issues':

New ways of working

- **'Boundary spanners'** – believe in collaboration, demonstrate an ability to obtain and distribute information strategically, see

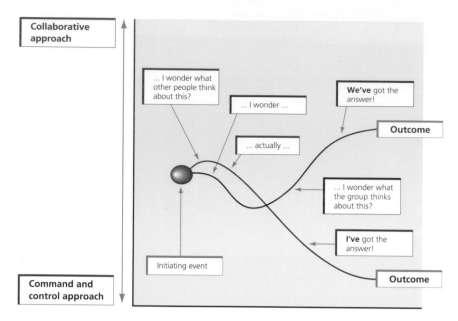

Figure 10.3 The leadership 'gap'. *Source*: Adapted from www.anecdote.com.au, accessed 30 June 2009.

problems in new ways, craft solutions, develop and support the others' skills (Bradshaw, 1999);

- **'Tempered radicals'** – willing to act on different external agendas and take risks, yet work successfully within organisations (Meyerson, 2004);
- **Broker, mediator and negotiator** – increasingly being recognised, recruited and trained for specific cross-boundary roles;
- Thinking differently about leadership and followership – professionals are rarely passive followers, people choose to follow, no one leads all the time. Skills of **active followership**, little 'l' leadership (leading in small ways, at all levels) and big 'L' leadership (leading from the front), are all as valuable as one another and need to be incorporated into the leadership repertoire (Kelley, 1992).

Collaborative strategies

Even when support for collaboration and partnership working is strong, shared initiatives are often imposed in a contractual and legalistic fashion. This can cause resistance. Understanding organisational and interpersonal barriers to collaboration and using knowledge and skills from both leadership and management

will facilitate cross-boundary and collaborative working. Activities might include

- raising your awareness of organisations' and professionals' responsibilities and powers;
- learning the systems, processes and ways of working (cultures) to identify and overcome structural and societal obstacles to collaboration;
- thinking of how funding mechanisms can be used across collaborations by aligning, pooling or disaggregating funds;
- stimulating cross-functional and organisational working through becoming involved in new projects or health innovations;
- using a project management approach to achieve a strong collaboration through a 'guiding coalition', stakeholder involvement, defining vision, mutual benefit (collaborative advantage) and visible wins;
- mapping systems and your connections with others to help identify networks through which change can be effected.

Collaborative clinical leaders need to work hard to identify and develop shared values between organisations, professions and communities. Above all, their leadership is not about personal glory

Table 10.2 Shared and collaborative leadership.

Characteristics	Heroic leadership	Shared and collaborative leadership
Is found:	At the top of organisations	Throughout organisations – a cadre of leaders
Decision and strategy is crafted by:	The top	Cadre of people who solve problems
Impact:	Holds and retains power	Helps others achieve their potential
Motivating others is based on:	Myth/mystique and charismatic authority Positional power	Collaborative engagement
Trust is found in:	Processes	Relationships Values
Change is:	Initiated by the top and resisted by those below	Initiated through development and innovation
Rewards mostly go to:	Shareholders, leaders and senior managers	All who help the organisation achieve improvements All stakeholders affected by the organisation's actions

Source: Adapted from Lee-Davis *et al.*, 2007.

but about making a real and lasting difference in healthcare delivery to the people and communities that engage in it (Table 10.2; Box 10.4).

Box 10.4 **Case study: Collaborative leadership**

A group of senior leaders from universities and health and social care organisations had been meeting informally to discuss ideas for a regional collaboration. The group took advantage of key drivers, including a policy paper on simulation, the need for all organisations to demonstrate efficiency in practice placements, the patient safety agenda, community mental health legislation and a willingness to collaborate. The group established a formal collaborative, devised a project bid, applied for funding from the Department of Health and initiated a new educational programme for health and social care professionals to work collaboratively in a simulated environment around clinical and professional decision-making for people with mental health issues.

Programmes were developed for undergraduate students, postgraduate students and continuing professional development for experienced practitioners. The impact on patient care through these interprofessional collaborations was measurable and influential, leading to the establishment of a national training programme for health and social care professionals using simulation.

References

Bradshaw L. Principals as boundary spanners: Working collaboratively to solve problems. *NASSP Bulletin* 1999; **83**(611): 38–47.

Department of Health. *Putting People First: A shared vision and commitment to the transformation of adult social care*. The Stationery Office, London. 2008.

Department of Health. *High Quality Care for All: The NHS Next Stage Review final report*. The Stationery Office, London. 2009.

Greenleaf RK. *Servant Leadership: A Journey into the Nature of Legitimate Power and Greatness*. Paulist Press, Mahwah, NJ. 1977.

Hartle F, Snook P, Apsey H, Browton R. The training and development of middle managers in the Children's Workforce. Report by the Hay Group to the Children's Workforce Development Council (CWDC). 2008, http://www.cwdcouncil.org.uk/assets/0000/2362/Training_and_development_of_middle_managers_in_the_children_s_workforce.pdf, accessed 22 July 2010.

Imison C, Giordano RW. Doctors as leaders. *British Medical Journal* 2009; **338**(7701): 979.

Kanter RM. The middle manager as innovator. *Harvard Business Review* 1982; **60**(4): 95–105.

Kelley RE. *The Power of Followership*. Doubleday, New York. 1992.

Laming H. *The Victoria Climbié Inquiry:* Report of an inquiry by Lord Laming. Cm 5730. The Stationery Office, London. 2003.

Lee-Davies L, Kakabadse NK, Kakabadse A. Shared leadership: Leading through polylogue. *Business Strategy Series* 2007; **8**(4): 246–53.

Lewin K. *Field Theory in Social Science: Selected theoretical papers*. D Cartwright (ed.). Harper & Row, New York. 1951.

Liedtka JM, Whitten E. Enhancing care delivery through cross-disciplinary collaboration: A case study. *Journal of Healthcare Management* 1998; **43**(2): 185–203.

McKimm J, Millard L, Held S. Leadership, education and partnership: Project LEAP: Developing educational regional leadership capacity in higher education and health services through collaboration and partnership working. *International Journal of Public Services Leadership* 2008; **4**(4): 24–48.

Meyerson D. The tempered radicals. *Stanford Social Innovation Review* 2004; **2**(2): 14–23.

Simkins T. *Leadership in education: 'What Works' or 'Makes Sense'?* Professorial lecture given at Sheffield Hallam University. 2004

Snowden DJ, Boone ME. A leader's framework for decision making. *Harvard Business Review* 2007; **85**(11): 68–76.

Wenger E. *Communities of Practice: Learning, Meaning and Identity*. Cambridge University Press, Cambridge. 1998.

World Health Organization. *Everybody's Business: Strengthening Health Systems to Improve Health Outcomes: WHO's Framework for Action*. WHO, Geneva. 2007.

World Health Organization. *Framework for Action on Interprofessional Education and Collaborative Practice*. WHO, Geneva. 2010.

Further resources

Baker D, Day R, Salas E. Teamwork as an essential component of high-reliability organisations. *HSR: Health Services Research* 2006; **41**(4, part 2): 1576–98.

Bolman LG, Deal T. *Reframing Organizations: Artistry, choice and leadership*, 3rd edn. Jossey-Bass, San Francisco. 2003.

Kouzes JM, Posner BZ. *The Leadership Challenge*. Jossey-Bass, San Francisco. 2003.

McKimm J, Phillips K (eds) *Leadership and Management in Integrated Services*. Learning Matters, Exeter. 2009.

CHAPTER 11

Understanding Yourself as Leader

Jennifer King

Edgecumbe Consulting Group Ltd, Bristol, UK

> **OVERVIEW**
>
> - 'Who we are is how we lead' (Hogan & Kaiser, 2004)
> - Personality has a significant influence on leadership effectiveness
> - Clinicians need to understand how traits that make them good clinicians may not serve them well as leaders – and vice versa
> - Leaders need to use their strengths to the full – but guard against over-playing their strengths, which may lead to 'derailment'
> - No single leader can be complete: good leaders use other team members to complement their traits, type and abilities
> - Leaders can develop and become more effective with the help of feedback and coaching

Personality and leadership

The most effective leaders are aware of their strengths and limitations and how these affect those they lead. Research has clearly shown a significant correlation between personality, leadership effectiveness and an organisation's performance (Figure 11.1). Personality alone does not, however, make a good or bad leader. Rather, it sets up predispositions for leaders to behave in certain ways – and these behaviours will either help or hinder the effectiveness of the leader. Furthermore, traits and behaviours that make clinicians good at the technical aspects of patient care may serve them less well in the arena of clinical leadership.

If clinicians can understand themselves and their impact on others, this self-awareness can be applied to developing themselves more effectively as clinical leaders – both playing to their strengths and recognising and avoiding potential pitfalls.

The 'ideal' leadership profile

Countless studies of leadership traits have sought to identify the 'perfect' leader profile. There is now a clear picture emerging of the

characteristics that are most likely to help or hinder effective leadership. Personality research over the last three decades has culminated in the identification of five key 'domains', known as the Big Five that, in various ways, significantly affect success at work, including effectiveness as a leader (Barrick & Mount, 1991); see Box 11.1. The constellation of personality traits that predicts success as a leader is as follows: emotional stability (resilience to stress and setbacks), extroversion (sociable, assertive and energetic), openness to experience (intellectually curious, adaptable to change and empathic) and conscientiousness (focused, organised and dutiful).

> Box 11.1 **The Big Five personality dimensions**
>
> **Neuroticism:** need for stability, emotional reactivity
> **Extroversion:** sociability, enthusiasm and activity
> **Openness:** originality, openness to experience
> **Agreeableness:** adaptability and cooperation
> **Conscientiousness:** will to achieve, focus, organise

As well as possessing certain personality traits, effective leaders need to be able to do five tasks: inspire people, focus their efforts, enable them to do their job, reinforce their efforts (managing both good and poor performance) and help them to learn. Personality may affect the extent to which a leader can or cannot carry out these tasks effectively. For example, highly conscientious leaders are likely to be better at focusing than leaders who are themselves unfocused or disorganised. Leaders who are agreeable are likely to be better at enabling and rewarding but less good at tackling poor performance.

The incomplete leader

No leader can be complete: it is rare for any individual leader to have the 'perfect' personality profile. Leaders who have strong skills with people may sacrifice some effectiveness in getting quick results, and vice versa. Leaders should therefore recognise others in their team who can complement the attributes and behaviours they lack. A clinical leader who finds conflict difficult will benefit from enrolling a more tough-minded colleague to handle difficult negotiations. A leader who is more pragmatic and more resistant to

---

ABC of Clinical Leadership, 1st edition.
Edited by Tim Swanwick and Judy McKimm. © 2011 Blackwell Publishing Ltd.

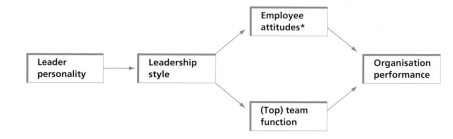

Figure 11.1 The links between leader personality and organisation performance.
*Including engagement. *Source*: Hogan & Kaiser, 2005.

change may need to draw on other more innovative team members. See Chapter 4 for more on leading teams.

Type and leadership

Each leader has a unique set of gifts which may help them in some situations and hinder them in others (Box 11.2). This is the premise of the well-known Myers-Briggs Type Inventory (MBTI; Kirby, 1997). Rather than identifying the type of characteristics that make a good leader, the MBTI highlights differences in type preferences (Box 11.3) and shows how these can affect leadership. Different ways of leading may have different implications for patient care. Effective leaders ensure that they appreciate and deploy the different gifts of those in their team(s). In our example, Anna is possibly a more introverted (I) leader who is less communicative and may need the help of a more extrovert colleague to present ideas. She also may be a (T), a logical leader who approaches difficult decisions with cool objectivity, but may need the guidance of a colleague who is more alert to the effect on others (F), in this case Fay. A more intuitive (N) leader may be good at taking a strategic approach but may need others with a better eye for detail (S). Were Fay and Anna to learn to appreciate and understand one another's personality styles, they might work more effectively with one another and as part of a team.

> Box 11.2 **Case study: Personality types**
>
> Fay is just coming to the end of her second foundation year and, although she feels she has done well in previous rotations and has had good feedback from colleagues and patients, she is struggling working with Anna, the lead consultant on the service. Fay finds Anna quite cold, with a brusque style and approach. Fay also feels that her way of working collaboratively through discussion with the wider multidisciplinary team and with patients (which was praised in other rotations) is not what her boss wants and Anna constantly criticises Fay for not making decisions fast enough. How might an understanding of personality types help Fay and Anna?

Being predisposed to a certain personality type does not prevent leaders from leading in certain ways, but it can make it more difficult. It means, for example, that a leader who is not naturally communicative can learn ways to improve, but development may be long and slow. Ultimately, a good leader will recognise and accept where changes can be made and where it may be more productive to call on others with complementary types.

> Box 11.3 **The dimensions of the Myers-Briggs Type Indicator**
>
> **Extroverts(E):** energised by people; talk their way through problems
>
> **Introverts (I):** energised by ideas; prefer time for reflection; may not express ideas openly
>
> **Sensors (S):** focus on data, facts, and the present
>
> **Intuitives (N):** focus on possibilities and the future; see the big picture
>
> **Thinkers (T):** make decisions based on objective data, logic
>
> **Feelers (F):** make decisions based on values, feelings
>
> **Judgers (J):** prefer to plan, be organised and structured; reach a conclusion
>
> **Perceivers (P):** prefer keeping options open; flexible, spontaneous, casual

The 'emotionally intelligent' leader

Effective leadership is more than simply being self-aware. It also requires being aware of the impact that you have on others and being able to manage this appropriately. Many clinical leaders are intelligent and effective in their technical field, but may be less 'emotionally intelligent' (Goleman, 1998). Emotional intelligence, known as EI (or EQ, as opposed to IQ), is now widely considered a core component of managerial and professional effectiveness (Box 3.1). There are now a number of strategies that clinical leaders can use to develop aspects of EI, through coaching and other support.

The leader and the team

Leader personality has a powerful effect on team functioning and team climate (how it feels to work in the team). It has been found that how employees view their supervisor is the primary determinant of their satisfaction. The personality of the leader plays a significant role.

Leaders who are emotionally sensitive and agreeable may be more likely to notice and act on signs of stress in their colleagues. They are also more likely to show appreciation and to accommodate people's needs. They need, however, to prevent their desire for acceptance and approval from hindering their willingness to handle conflict.

Leaders who are more *dis*agreeable – more competitive, sceptical, and even antagonistic – may be well-equipped to make controversial decisions or tackle under-performance, without fear of disapproval. Such leaders can often achieve significant results in terms of delivery of targets or driving up performance standards.

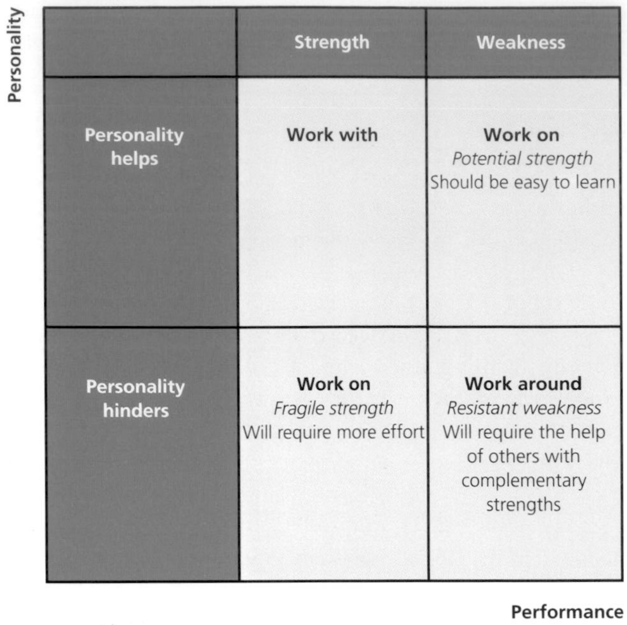

Figure 11.2 Working with, on or around your personality.

They are likely to respond well in a crisis when immediate results or action are required. However, their tough-minded style can have short-term pay-offs and may be less likely to engage and motivate team members over the longer-term.

Can leaders change their personality and style?

Since personality tends to remain stable over time, there may be little that you as a leader can do to change your underlying traits or type. But by becoming aware of what you do well or less well, and then understanding how your personality may help or hinder you in these areas (Figure 11.2), you can focus their development more productively, as follows:

- Decide which areas of your leadership performance you are good at and less good at.
- Consider how your personality helps and hinders you in these areas. These will be the traits that predispose you to certain types of behaviour.
- Identify what you need to work with, on or around to make the most of your traits and abilities.

For example, you may have learnt to be a good team builder (a strength). However, if you are introvert and not naturally sociable, your personality may hinder you in this area. Good team building, for you, is likely to require continued effort. Others may not appreciate how difficult this is for you. This means you need to keep working on it to keep up your competence. If, however, you have never been much good at team working (a weakness) and your personality is also a hindrance, any possible improvement is likely to be time-consuming and frustrating. So a work-around solution may be required: enlisting the help of someone who is more of a natural team builder and working closely with them.

Leadership 'derailers'

Leadership effectiveness is not just a matter of having enough of 'the right stuff', it is also a matter of not having too much of 'the wrong stuff'. Poor leadership is not just an absence of technical skills. Research clearly shows that flawed interpersonal skills can undermine a leader's effectiveness as well as the performance of their team (e.g. Goleman, 1998).

The attributes for which many leaders are valued and that contribute to their achievements are invariably the same characteristics that may be responsible for their downfall. When leaders are exposed to particular stress or pressure, for example the transition to a new role, pressure to deliver results or to build a new team, they may over-play some of their natural strengths to the point of becoming counter-productive. Thus strengths become weaknesses and, ultimately, lead to dysfunctional behaviour.

Hogan and Hogan (2001) identify 11 such personality derailers (Box 11.4). Leaders must learn to recognise and manage their own particular derailing characteristics, so that they can continue to exercise their strengths without allowing these to become counter-productive.

Box 11.4 **Leadership 'derailers'**	
Strength	**Associated weakness ('dark side' emerging under pressure)**
Enthusiastic	Volatile: unpredictable, volatile
Careful	Cautious: indecisive, risk-averse
Shrewd	Mistrustful: vindictive
Independent	Detached: withdrawn, uncommunicative
Focused	Passive-aggressive: stubborn, fixed on own agenda
Confident	Arrogant: entitled, opinionated, won't admit mistakes
Charming	Manipulative: tests limits, takes risks, defies rules
Vivacious	Dramatic: histrionic, attention-seeking
Imaginative	Eccentric: erratic, unusual, fanciful
Diligent	Perfectionist: rigid, over-controlling
Dutiful	Dependent: indecisive, overly keen for approval from seniors

Source: Hogan & Hogan, 2001.

In the clinical professions, this may be evidenced in minor day-to-day occurrences, but it also may underlie some of the major failures to care for patients. Box 11.5 lists some excerpts from the summary report into the Bristol Inquiry into the management of care of children receiving complex cardiac surgical services at the Bristol Royal Infirmary between 1984 and 1995 (Department of Health, 2001). The report criticised much about the management systems, leadership and culture at Bristol and, as you read the excerpts, consider whether the personality 'derailers' described above and lack of self-insight may have played a part in what occurred over a number of years in a busy pressured environment.

Derailment can be prevented through timely feedback that alerts the leader when his or her behaviour has crossed the line into unacceptable or dysfunctional behaviour. Such behaviour is, in effect, a response to stress; therefore it can also be prevented by effective stress management.

Box 11.5 **Case study: Learning from Bristol (2)**

It is an account of people who cared greatly about human suffering, and were dedicated and well-motivated. Sadly, some lacked insight and their behaviour was flawed. Many failed to communicate with each other, and to work together effectively for the interests of their patients. There was a lack of leadership, and of teamwork.

It is an account of a hospital where there was a 'club culture'; an imbalance of power, with too much control in the hands of a few individuals.

What was unusual about Bristol was that the systems and culture in place were such as to make open discussion and review more difficult. Staff were not encouraged to share their problems or to speak openly. Those who tried to raise concerns found it hard to have their voice heard.

The evidence of parents was mixed. To some, the staff, doctors, nurses and others were dedicated and caring and could not have done more. To others, some staff were helpful while others were not. To others again, the staff, largely the doctors and particularly the surgeons, were uncaring and they misled parents.

The quality of healthcare would be enhanced by a greater degree of respect and honesty in the relationship between healthcare professional and patient. Good communication is essential, but as the Royal College of Surgeons of England told us:

' ... it is the area of greatest compromise in the practices of most surgeons in the NHS and the source of most complaints'.

Medical schools must ensure that the criteria for selecting future doctors include the potential to be versatile, flexible and sensitive. They must also ensure that healthcare professionals are not drawn from too narrow an academic and socio-economic base.

Source: Department of Health, 2001.

Developing as a leader

How do leaders stay on track, and manage their traits – both helpful and unhelpful – to sustain a high level of effectiveness? Feedback is crucial. The Emperor's New Clothes is the salutary tale of a leader who ignored – or worse, discouraged – feedback. When someone was brave enough to speak up and draw the Emperor's attention to his failings, the damage had already been done. Leaders need to be open to feedback, encourage a climate where feedback is given constructively and regularly and to seek regular input from trusted colleagues. This can be done opportunistically (e.g. before or after a difficult meeting) or more formally through multi-source (360 degree) feedback surveys from a range of colleagues and patients.

Coaching can be particularly effective as a means of helping leaders to manage these areas of behaviour, particularly if it is preceded with a full assessment of the leader's personality and capabilities (Nelson & Hogan, 2009). Not only does this help development to become more targeted and tailored to the individual leader; it also helps to ensure that the coaching itself is approached in the most effective way, for example leaders who are emotionally volatile may start off enthusiastically and quickly become discouraged. Leaders who are over-confident, perhaps even a little narcissistic, may resist any hint of critical feedback. A skilled coach can help the leader to recognise how these characteristics may play out in the workplace.

Clinicians as leaders

Leadership presents a particular challenge for clinicians. Most healthcare professionals are motivated by a strong desire to help and care for patients. They are often, by nature, highly agreeable. This trait is more likely to make a good clinician but not necessarily a good leader. Leaders are more challenging: they encourage others to change. They may have to tackle conflict, or push hard for resources. Therefore, many clinicians who seek to lead may find themselves working against their natural, altruistic traits, and instead are having to learn ways to be tougher and more single-minded about delivering change and improvements to patient care (Pendleton, 2002). This may at times bring them into direct conflict with their values and personal disposition. Whilst this may not always be avoided, understanding when and why such conflicts occur can prove valuable in seeking strategies to manage them.

Most importantly, there is evidence that effective leadership can have real benefits to patient care (Firth-Cozens, 2006). Therefore, understanding what underpins your behaviour as a clinical leader and using this to develop your role will help to ensure that you are using your leadership abilities to the full.

References

Barrick MR, Mount MK. The Big Five personality dimensions and job performance: A meta-analysis. *Personnel Psychology* 1991; **44**: 1–26.

Department of Health. *Learning from Bristol: The Report of the Public Inquiry into Children's Heart Surgery at the Bristol Royal Infirmary 1984–1995.* The Stationery Office, London. 2001.

Firth-Cozens J. Leadership and the quality of care. In: J Cox, J King, A Hutchinson, P McAvoy (eds), *Understanding Doctors' Performance.* Radcliffe Medical Press, Abingdon. 2006.

Goleman D. *Working with Emotional Intelligence.* Bloomsbury, London. 1998.

Hogan R, Hogan J. Assessing leadership: A view from the dark side. *International Journal of Selection and Assessment* 2001; **9**: 40–51.

Hogan R, Kaiser RB. What we know about leadership. *Review of General Psychology* 2005; **9**(2): 169–80.

Kirby LK. Psychological type and the Myers-Briggs Type Indicator. In: C Fitzgerald, LK Kirby (eds), *Developing Leaders: Research and Applications in Psychological Type and Leadership Development.* Davies-Black Publishing, Palo Alto, CA. 1997.

Nelson E, Hogan R. Coaching on the dark side. *International Coaching Psychology Review* 2009; **4**(1): 9–21.

Pendleton DA. *Our values.* Paper presented at the Royal College of General Practitioners' 50th Anniversary Celebration, Birmingham. 2002.

Further resources

Howard PJ, Howard MJ. *The Owner's Manual for Personality at Work.* Centre for Applied Cognitive Studies, Charlotte, NC. 2001.

Acknowledgements

The author acknowledges the contribution of Dr David Pendleton, of the Edgecumbe Consulting Group, to this chapter.

CHAPTER 12

Leading in a Culturally Diverse Health Service

Tim Swanwick[1] and Judy McKimm[2]

[1]London Deanery, London, UK
[2]Unitec, Auckland, New Zealand

OVERVIEW

- Healthcare workforces and patient populations are increasingly culturally diverse
- Addressing diversity and equality is key to ensuring effective healthcare delivery
- Effective clinical leaders demonstrate cultural competence and understand how cultural factors impact on service delivery and health outcomes
- An understanding of the legal framework underpinning diversity and equality is important
- Attending to cultural factors in the workplace can help reduce clinical errors and improve patient safety

Introduction

In their book and interactive planning process *Future Search*, Weisbord and Janoff (2010) describe a historical trend in the leadership of improvement culminating in 'everybody' being involved in whole system reform (Box 12.1). This resonates strongly with the concept of distributed leadership discussed in Chapter 3. Diversity is needed within a system to allow for future evolution; but not everyone has an equal opportunity to get involved, owing to a range of factors, including the impact of cultural background and the perceptions of others.

Clinical leaders need to appreciate the norms and values of different cultures and understand how they perceive leadership and its associated behaviours. Such an understanding will enable more effective leadership (and followership) practices and, as a result, the delivery of more culturally sensitive and appropriate patient care.

What is diversity?

Diversity is about recognising individual and group differences and valuing the contributions of everyone in society. The 'diversity agenda' covers issues such as personality, class, professional background, educational attainment, gender, disability, sexual orientation, age and ethnicity. Equality, on the other hand, is about 'creating a fairer society, where everyone can participate and has the opportunity to fulfil their potential' (Department of Health, 2004). An equalities approach identifies patterns of experience based on group identity and the processes that limit an individual's health and life chances. In terms of occupational disparities, for example, people from black and minority ethnic groups comprise 39.1% of NHS hospital medical staff but only 22.1% of all hospital medical consultants (Department of Health, 2005).

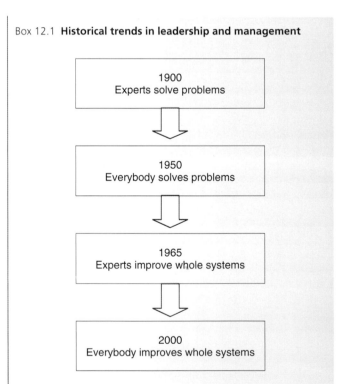

Box 12.1 **Historical trends in leadership and management**

Jehn *et al.* (1999) describe three types of diversity:

- social category: concerned with demographic differences;
- informational: concerned with knowledge, education, experience;
- value: personality and attitudes.

In this chapter we focus on social category diversity, and in particular cultural diversity in relation to issues of race and ethnicity.

ABC of Clinical Leadership, 1st edition.
Edited by Tim Swanwick and Judy McKimm. © 2011 Blackwell Publishing Ltd.

Diversity within healthcare systems

The environment in which healthcare is delivered, and the workforce responsible for its delivery, is increasingly culturally diverse. In the United Kingdom, the proportion of population from ethnic minority backgrounds rose from 7.3% in 2000 to 10.3% in 2007. This trend is set to continue with, at the time of writing, ethnic minorities comprising 17% of undergraduates and 20% of pupils in state-funded schools.

Against this background, the NHS – an employer where 15% of current employees are from black and ethnic minorities – views proactively managing diversity as critical to its success by

- promoting the NHS as the employer of choice;
- recruiting a workforce that meets capacity and delivery needs;
- increasing productivity through maximising individual contributions to patient care;
- protecting trusts from litigation.

(NHS Employers, 2009)

As healthcare systems become more closely tailored to the needs of patients, delivered locally and integrated across services, it is essential that clinical leaders understand cultural differences to identify areas where targeted action is needed. In Box 12.2 we have listed some common situations that require different approaches to healthcare delivery for people from different cultures.

Box 12.2 **Situations requiring acknowledgement of cultural diversity**

- Illness behaviour
- Attitudes to nudity
- Birth rituals
- Birth control
- Blood transfusions
- Involvement of carer or family in decision-making
- Clothing and dress norms
- Concepts of sickness, healing and care
- Disability and rehabilitation
- Language and translation requirements
- Palliative care, preparation for death, dying and death rituals
- Preferences for practitioner gender or culture

Source: Queensland Government, 2009.

A key leadership challenge for those managing health services is that migration patterns resulting from increased employment mobility and shifting political and economic landscapes mean that many health workforces are not only increasingly culturally diverse but are also more transient. In rural, remote and deprived areas, which often have large ethnic minority populations, recruiting and retaining doctors and other health professionals is particularly challenging. A range of educational and service interventions have been established to train and attract staff to underserved areas, specifically staff from similar backgrounds to local populations. But interventions have to be lawful and need to demonstrate cultural safety (see the following section on legislative frameworks). These

may include affirmative or positive action programmes for entry to medical school or recruitment of staff from a specific ethnic group. Positive action (Box 12.3) is being promoted at all levels in UK health services, including the identification of future black and ethnic minority leaders, as evidenced by the NHS 'Breaking Through' programme (www.nhsbreakingthrough.co.uk).

Box 12.3 **Positive action**

Positive action is a range of lawful action that seeks to address an imbalance in employment opportunities among targeted groups that have previously experienced disadvantage or that have been subject to discriminatory policies and practices or that are underrepresented in the workforce.

Source: NHS Employers, 2005.

In the United States, many healthcare providers have established specific cultural initiatives aimed at improving healthcare. One example is Kaiser Permanente, which has implemented a number of interventions, such as culturally targeted healthcare delivery where the majority of staff members are recruited on the basis of cultural background and capabilities; onsite interpreting services; and a national director of linguistic and cultural programmes. These interventions have led not only to quality improvements and the reduction of racial/ethnic disparities but also to more productive health services (Betancourt *et al.*, 2002).

Legislative frameworks

Clinical leaders and managers need to understand the legal basis for equality and diversity and be able to apply this in practice. UK legislation has two main elements (Table 12.1): the anti-discriminatory framework, which gives individuals a route to raise complaints of discrimination around employment and service delivery, and public duties, which place a proactive duty on organisations to address institutional discrimination (Webb & McKimm, 2007). Discrimination is described as where someone is treated less favourably or poorly because of one or more aspects of their social identity. Public duties apply to all public bodies, including national health services, NHS Trusts and bodies and educational establishments.

Cultural competence and cultural safety

Cultural competence has been defined as the ability of individuals to look beyond their own cultural interpretations, to maintain objectivity when dealing with individuals from other cultures and to demonstrate an ability to understand behaviours without passing judgement (Bhugra & Americano, 2007). In healthcare it has been defined as 'the routine application of culturally appropriate health care interventions and practices' (Wells, 2000). The concept of 'cultural safety' (Ramsden, 1992) describes a safe environment where 'there is no assault, challenge or denial of a person's identity of who they are and what they need ... The people most able or equipped to provide a culturally safe atmosphere are people

Table 12.1 Overview of UK legal framework.

Anti-discriminatory		
Legislation	**Key legal principles**	**Who is protected**
Sex Discrimination Act 1975 Race Relations Act 1976 Disability Discrimination Act 1995 Employment Equality (Sexual Orientation) and (Religious Belief) Regulations 2003 Employment Equality (Age) Regulations 2006 Equality Act 2006 (Covers service delivery in relation to sexual orientation and religious belief) Equality Bill 2009 (Includes age legislation in the area of employment and service delivery and strengthens requirements to promote equality) The SEN and Disability Act 2001 (This Act extended the Disability Discrimination Act 1995 to education and training with effect from September 2002. This act requires teachers to explore the provision of reasonable adjustments for students who may have disabilities, including learning disabilities, to enable them to participate effectively.)	• Direct and indirect discrimination • Harassment • Reasonable adjustment • Positive action • Genuine Occupational Qualification • Victimisation	**Gender** women, men, people in relation to gender reassignment **Sexuality** lesbians, gay men, bisexual, transgender and heterosexual people **Race/ethnicity** anyone, where ethnic origin, colour or culture are concerned **Religion/belief** anyone, where religious or philosophical belief, including not having a particular religion or belief, is concerned **Disability** anyone who considers that they have an impairment that has a substantial and long-term effect on their ability to carry out day-to-day duties **Age** anyone of any age

Public duties		
Legislation	**General requirements on organisations**	**Specific requirements on organisations**
Race Relations Amendment Act 2000 Disability Discrimination Act 2005 Equality Act 2006	Produce a (race, disability and gender) equality scheme Carry out impact assessments on their functions, policies and practices Carry out equalities monitoring and take action to address any imbalance Publish the results of any work undertaken	**All groups:** Promote equality of opportunity **Gender:** Ensure that they do not discriminate unlawfully between women and men when carrying out employment or service functions **Race/ethnicity:** Eliminate unlawful discrimination **Disability:** Eliminate unlawful discrimination

Source: Adapted from Webb & McKimm, 2007.

from the same culture' (Williams, 1999). The concepts of cultural competence and safety provide a basis for embedding culturally appropriate health, employment and education practices, enhancing personal empowerment and improving service delivery. Boyer (2003) argues that the World Health Organization and United Nations declarations on the right to health encompass the right to a culturally appropriate healthcare system. This includes the right to access different forms of treatment (such as traditional medicine or healing practices) and the right for self-determination (Stout & Downey, 2006). Inequalities in healthcare resulting from cultural factors may then need to be addressed at many levels: societal, organisational, professional and interpersonal.

The culturally competent clinical leader

At the interpersonal level, culturally competent leadership involves a similar skill set as culturally competent patient care. Many of the issues are the same and relate to understanding, empathy, sense-making and motivation coupled with shared respect, meaning, knowledge and experience, of learning together with dignity, and truly listening.

Berlin and Fowkes (1983) propose a simple model (LEARN) for consultations in family practice, adapted here for leadership:

• **Listen** – and seek to understand the perspectives of others
• **Explain** – your perceptions and strategies
• **Acknowledge** – and discuss differences and similarities
• **Recommend** – a way forward while remembering cultural parameters
• **Negotiate** – an agreement that respects prevailing cultural frameworks

As well as demonstrating respect and empathy, leaders need to be able to challenge discrimination or unlawful practice. This requires an understanding of the legal framework and the rights of different groups as well as the personal courage and capacity to challenge poor practice at individual and organisational levels (Table 12.2).

Thomas and Ely (1996) suggest that leaders who want to manage diversity effectively need to move away from the traditional paradigms of *discrimination and fairness* (as enshrined in legislation) towards *access and legitimacy* (which accept and celebrate difference). They suggest a new paradigm which actively connects

Table 12.2 Culturally competent leadership.

Be aware of:	Example
Assumptions and cultural stereotypes	It is important not to make assumptions about an individual's nationality and background based on skin colour or other visual cues (e.g. dress)
Formal and informal community support networks	Find ways of engaging community groups and patient representatives in healthcare decision-making Ask patients/carers about their cultural preferences
The cultural web and shadow side of organisations	Think about workplace culture (e.g. a long-hours culture that favours those without domestic responsibilities; where do 'corridor conversations' take place - who is involved and who is excluded?)
Language and communication	Is the message getting through (e.g. 12% of US citizens' first language is not English)? Challenge idiomatic or idiosyncratic use of language, including jargon
Influence of religion and spirituality	Providing time and space for religious needs and rights, e.g. daily prayers, acceptance of headwear, acknowledging holidays or Sabbaths when planning rotas
Institutional racism, harassment or discrimination	Raise awareness of what these mean, what the law says and people's employment and service rights. When it goes wrong, it can be both distressing and expensive
Habits, customs, behaviours or beliefs	Insensitivity can cause friction (e.g. think about dietary needs or specific cultural practices, such as prayers, blessings, hand washing, when planning events or meetings that provide food)
Educational level and employment experiences	Professional qualifications and experience may not translate from one country to another so don't make assumptions and try to spot talent (e.g. cardiologists working as taxi drivers). Be aware of alternative routes to professional practice and challenge inequitable systems
Migration experience	Be aware that before fleeing from war or oppression and becoming refugees, people came from all socioeconomic backgrounds, with standing and respect from their own communities – this is often lost when they emigrate or flee
Socioeconomic status	Consider whether people can afford to participate in out-of-work activities and events; think about challenging pay disparities

diversity to approaches to work: *the learning and effectiveness paradigm*. This approach incorporates and integrates all employees' perspectives into work processes and links closely to the emerging patient empowerment, personalisation and community-orientated approaches to public services we have discussed elsewhere.

Thomas and Ely suggest there are eight preconditions for making this paradigm shift, and these are summarised in Box 12.4.

Box 12.4 **Making the paradigm shift from *discrimination* and *fairness* to *access* and *legitimacy***

1. Leadership must understand that a diverse workforce will embody different perspectives and approaches to work and must truly value opinion and insight.
2. The leadership must recognise both the learning opportunities and the challenges that the expression of different perspectives presents for an organisation – leadership must be committed to persevering during the long period of learning and relearning.
3. The organisational culture must create an expectation of high standards of performance from everyone, and not expect less from some employees than others; such negative assumptions can lead to self-fulfilling prophecies.
4. The organisational culture must stimulate personal development through careful job design, training and education.
5. The organisational culture must encourage openness, enabling a high tolerance for debate and supporting constructive conflict on work-related matters.
6. The culture must make employees feel valued, encouraging commitment and empowerment.
7. The organisation must have a well-articulated and well-understood mission which maintains a focal point centred on the accomplishment of goals.

---

8. The organisation must have a relatively egalitarian, non-bureaucratic structure that promotes the exchange of ideas and welcomes constructive challenges to 'the way we do things round here'. Leaders need to separate the enabling elements of bureaucracy (the ability to get things done) from the disabling elements (those that create resistance to experimentation).

Source: Thomas & Ely, 1996.

Cultural variation in leadership practices

Hofstede (2001) points out that, although cultures differ, they all meet the same five basic problems of social life: identity, hierarchy and power distance, gender, truth and virtue. An awareness of this can empower and enable individuals to lead and manage more effectively.

Different cultures adopt different positions on a spectrum of social participation between *individualism* and *communitarianism*. According to Hampden-Turner and Trompenaars (2000), individualism is characterised by competition, self-reliance, self-interest and personal growth and fulfilment, whereas communitarianism (equated with socio-centrism or collectivism) relies on social concern, altruism, cooperation, public service and societal legacy. Extremes at both ends of the scale can be destructive in organisations.

One of the largest studies into leadership practices across the world is the GLOBE project, which set out 'to determine the extent to which the practices and values of business leadership are universal and the extent to which they are specific to just a few societies' (House *et al.*, 2004).

Among the many and interesting findings of the project, which ran over 11 years across 62 countries, were six 'culturally endorsed

Table 12.3 Two culturally specific leadership styles.

Arabic	Anglo
1. Self-protective	1. Charismatic/values-based
2. Humane-orientated	2. Participative
3. Autonomous	3. Humane-orientated
4. Charismatic/values-based	4. Team-orientated
5. Team-orientated	5. Autonomous
6. Participative	6. Self-protective

Six 'culturally endorsed leadership theory dimensions' reflecting the essential ways in which middle managers worldwide distinguish between effective and ineffective leadership.
Source: House *et al.*, 2004.

leadership theory dimensions' or leadership styles that were weighted differently across nine geographical clusters. Table 12.3 provides an example of the differences between a rank ordering of an Anglo-cluster (UK/US) and an Arabic cluster. The implications here could be that Arabic leadership style may be more concerned with status, position and security whilst the Anglo style values participation more. Each list is presented in order of preference assigned by different cultural groups.

Box 12.5 **Case study: Leading for diversity**

Abra is the lead community midwife working in a primary care trust with a large Muslim population. It is a community of women with a poor obstetric record characterised by late presentations and antenatal complications, and is a source of frequent cultural and linguistic misunderstandings. She decides to address this by assembling an 'expert panel' of women from the local community. The panel meets with the community team in a workshop format to discuss their ideas, concerns and expectations in relation to pregnancy, childbirth and child-rearing. As a result, the team feels more empowered in supporting this group through their experiences of childbirth and later reports much more effective relationships and antenatal care. The women are pleased to have been consulted and keen to continue to be involved in the ongoing education of healthcare professionals. The panel becomes an established feature of the healthcare landscape and is subsequently asked for its input on a number of service redesign issues relating to local maternity and children's services.

Why does an understanding of such cultural differences matter? We can turn to the aviation industry for an example. Hofstede's work has been applied to some major air crashes, and research findings reveal that behind many air crashes lie failures of communication, including those stemming from the relationship between the captain and co-pilots (Helmreich & Merritt, 2000). Where more junior staff feel that the leader is above them in the social hierarchy (e.g. in the Korean Air crashes in the 1990s), their deference and unwillingness to challenge authority can lead to disaster. Discomfort with ambiguity can lead to teams sticking with procedure where a more flexible approach to uncertainty may help avoid risk. In the clinical context, Bleakley's (2006) and Lingard *et al.*'s (2004) research on social identity in the operating theatre and intensive care unit indicates that communication failures (including failure to engage in briefings or to speak out when something is wrong) and assumptions and behaviours based on cultural background

put patient safety at risk and increases clinical errors. The expectations followers have of their leaders varies greatly between cultures. Greater attention to developing good, clear, open communication between teams and professional groups is a key aim of culturally competent leaders (Box 12.5).

Conclusion

Culturally competent clinical leaders need to understand the communities they serve, the socio-cultural influences on individuals' health practices and beliefs and an understanding of the elements of health and social care systems that prevent certain groups from receiving quality healthcare. They need to devise strategies to reduce and monitor barriers to employment, education and training and healthcare that need to be adopted at the organisational level, the systemic level and in the clinical context. Effective strategies include positive action programmes to encourage leaders from under-represented groups into senior posts and involving communities in decisions and policy-making, providing language support and training students and staff in cross-cultural communication. What is encouraging in the UK health sector is a growing recognition of the need to value and respond to diversity issues. One important example of this is the commitment found in the Department of Health's policy document *Inspiring Leaders: Leadership for quality* (Department of Health, 2009) which states that all Strategic Health Authorities will have as one of their five-year outcomes:

an increased leadership supply, including clinical leaders, with leaders reflecting the workforce and the communities they serve (particularly people from black and minority ethnic backgrounds, women and disabled people).

And it is todays' healthcare leaders that are charged with turning the rhetoric into reality.

References

Berlin EA, Fowkes WC. A teaching framework for cross-cultural care. *West Journal of Medicine* 1983; **139**: 934–8.

Betancourt JR, Green AR, Carrillo JE. Cultural Competence in Health Care: Emerging Frameworks and Practical Approaches. 2002, http://www.commonwealthfund.org/~/media/Files/Publications/Fund%20Report/2002/Oct/Cultural%20Competence%20in%20Health%20Care%20%20Emerging%20Frameworks%20and%20Practical%20Approaches/betancourt_culturalcompetence_576%20pdf.pdf, accessed 19 July 2010.

Bhugra D, Americano A. Dealing with diversity. In: T Swanwick (ed.), *Understanding Medical Education* (series). Association for the Study of Medical Education, Edinburgh. 2007.

Bleakley A. You are who I say you are: The rhetorical construction of identity in the operating theatre. *Journal of Workplace Learning* 2006; **18**(7/8): 414–25.

Boyer Y. *The International Right to Health for Indigenous Peoples in Canada.* National Aboriginal Health Organization/The Native Law Centre, Ottawa/Saskatchewan. 2003.

Department of Health. *Sharing the Challenge, Sharing the Benefits: Equality and Diversity in the Medical Workforce Directorate.* Department of Health, London. 2004.

Department of Health. *Promoting Equality and Human Rights in the NHS: A Guide for Non-executive Directors of Boards.* Department of Health, London. 2005.

Department of Health. *Inspiring Leaders: Leadership for Quality: Guidance for NHS Talent and Leadership Plans*. Department of Health, London. 2009.

Hampden-Turner C, Trompenaars F. *Building Cross-cultural Competence*. Yale University Press, New Haven, CT. 2000.

Helmreich RL, Merritt A. Culture in the cockpit: Do Hoftstede's dimensions replicate? *Journal of Cross-Cultural Psychology* 2000; **31**(3): 283–301.

Hofstede, GJ. *Culture's Consequences: Comparing Values, Behaviours, Institutions and Organisations across Nations*. Sage, Thousand Oaks, CA. 2001.

House RJ, Hanges PJ, Javidan M *et al.* (eds) *Culture, Leadership and Organizations: The GLOBE Study of 62 Societies*. Sage, Thousand Oaks, CA. 2004.

Jehn KA, Northcraft GB, Neale MA. Why differences make a difference: A field study of diversity, conflict and performance in work groups. *Administrative Science Quarterly* 1999; **44**(4): 741–63.

Lingard L, Espin S, Evams C, Hawryluck L. The rules of the game: Interprofessional collaboration on the intensive care unit team. *Critical Care* 2004; **8**(6): R403–R408.

NHS Employers. *Positive action in the NHS*. Briefing Issue 10. 2005, http://www.nhsemployers.org/Aboutus/Publications/Documents/postive_action_briefing_10_151005.pdf, accessed 20 July 2010.

NHS Employers. *Managing Diversity: Making it Core Business*. NHS Employers, London. 2009, http://www.nhsemployers.org/Aboutus/Publications/Documents/Briefing_60_Managing_diversity_making_it_core_business.pdf, accessed 26 August 2009.

Queensland Government. Cultural Diversity. 2009, www.health.qld.gov.au/sop/content/cultural_diversity.asp, accessed 27 August 2009.

Ramsden IM. Cultural safety in nursing education in Aotearoa, presented at the Year of Indigenous Peoples Conference, Brisbane. 1992.

Stout MD, Downey B. Nursing indigenous peoples and cultural safety: So what? Now what? *Contemporary Nurse* 2006; **22**(2): 327–32.

Thomas DA, Ely RJ. Making differences matter: A new paradigm for managing diversity. *Harvard Business Review* 1996;**Sept/Oct**: 79–91.

Webb H, McKimm J. Diversity, Equal Opportunities and Human Rights. 2007, http://www.faculty.londondeanery.ac.uk/e-learning/diversity-equal-opportunities-and-human-rights, accessed 19 July 2010.

Weisbord M, Janoff S. *Future Search: An Action Guide to Finding Common Ground in Organizations and Communities*, Berrett-Koehler Publishers, San Francisco. 2010.

Wells MI. Beyond cultural competence: A model for individual and institutional cultural development. *Journal of Community Health Nursing* 2000; **17**(4): 189–99.

Williams R. Cultural safety: What does it mean for our work practice? *Australia and New Zealand Journal of Public Health* 1999; **23**(2): 212–14.

Further resources

Department of Health. Positively diverse: The field book: A practical guide to managing diversity in the NHS. 2001, http://www.dh.gov.uk/prod_consum_dh/groups/dh_digitalassets/@dh/@en/documents/digitalasset/dh_4074471.pdf, accessed 20 July 2010.

Department of Health. Equality, Diversity and Human Rights. 2010, http://www.dh.gov.uk/en/Managingyourorganisation/Equalityandhumanrights/index.htm, accessed 21 July 2010.

Equality and Human Rights Commission, http://www.equalityhumanrights.com/, accessed 21 July 2010.

Hofstede GJ, Pedersen PB, Hofstede G. *Exploring Culture: Exercises, Stories and Syntheticultures*. Intercultural Press, Yarmouth, ME. 2002.

Kandola R, Fullerton J. *Diversity in Action: Managing the Mosaic*. CIPD, London. 1998.

CHAPTER 13

Gender and Leadership

Beverly Alimo-Metcalfe[1] and Myfanwy Franks[2]

[1] Bradford University School of Management, and Real World Group, Leeds, UK
[2] Freelance Research Consultant, UK

OVERVIEW

- Leadership and culture are inextricably linked
- Notions of leadership, and the received wisdom on leadership, are gendered and this has implications on how it is assessed
- Heroic leadership is outdated and inappropriate for the NHS
- As organisational challenges grow in complexity and resources to deal with them diminish, embedding a culture of 'engagement' in healthcare organisations becomes paramount
- Research in the NHS shows that 'engaging leadership' predicts team effectiveness, staff morale and well-being, and that this approach is more likely to be adopted by women

The link between leadership and culture

Research has consistently shown that the most important contributor to organisational culture is the behaviour of those in leadership roles and, in particular, those in the most senior positions. The link between leadership and culture is inextricable: there is constant interplay between the two. Moreover, the most important responsibility of a leader is to create the appropriate culture.

The nature of leadership research

Notions of leadership have changed over time, as have definitions of what leadership is about, affected by social, technological, economic, and political change. What has been consistent, however, is that research into leadership has been dominated by US research, and most of this research has been about men, studying men, but the findings have been applied to humanity in general. Questions to ask when adopting a critical approach to the subject are listed in Box 13.1.

Are there gender differences in leadership?

Prior to the 1990s, few gender differences in leadership style were found, and when they were, they were relatively minor, but they generally suggested that women were likely to be more participative

and democratic in decision-making. When such differences were observed, however, the women's behaviour was not valued in its own right but was treated as a deviation (from the masculine norm) rather like a pathology that could be rectified by appropriate 'socialisation', such as attendance at an assertiveness course.

Box 13.1 Questions to ask when taking a critical approach to understanding models of leadership

1. Who funded the research on which it is based?
2. When did the research take place?
3. Where did it take place (e.g. country, culture)?
4. What major factors (e.g. economic, social) were influencing notions of leadership at the time?
5. What were the characteristics of the sample(s) studied, on whom the model was based (e.g. size, gender, ethnic and cultural background, type of organisation, level of 'leader', range of occupational groups studied)?
6. Is the model based on 'distant' leaders, such as famous CEOs or military leaders from history, or on 'nearby' leaders, such as immediate line managers?
7. Were the target 'leaders' defined as such by virtue of occupying a formal leadership position or were they defined as 'leaders' because the individuals had a particular impact on those they 'led'? In other words, is 'leadership' regarded as an independent variable or a dependent variable?
8. What was the methodology employed (e.g. case studies of individuals occupying top positions in organisations; gathering self-report data from the 'leaders' being studied, such as in interviews; or from soliciting views of leadership, from those who are 'led' by, or work with, the 'leaders')?

Other studies focused on whether there were gender differences in how men and women, in general, construe leadership. Women were found to construe leadership in more transformational terms, for example displaying more concern for empowering and involving others in decisions, whereas men, in general, perceived leadership in more transactional/agentic ways (Table 13.1).

Studies comparing men and women managers on transformational and transactional styles have found that women are more likely than men are to be rated, by their staff anonymously in 360-feedback processes, as more transformational – a style which is regarded as more effective than the transactional.

ABC of Clinical Leadership, 1st edition.
Edited by Tim Swanwick and Judy McKimm. © 2011 Blackwell Publishing Ltd.

Table 13.1 Male and female constructs of leadership.

Male constructs	Female constructs
• Gives clear directions	• Relates to others on an equal level
• Confident	• Strong and supportive
• Career-driven	• Concerned to take people with them
• Clarity of purpose	• Recognises delivery relies on others
• Organised	• Self-aware
• Analytical	• Honest with own values
• Politically skilled	

Source: Data collected from a sample of $n = 50$ senior female and male managers in the NHS using the repertory grid technique of interviewing.

What are the implications of gender differences for leadership behaviours?

If there are gender differences in 'implicit theories of leadership', that is in notions of what is appropriate leadership behaviour, and if one particular sex tends to dominate senior positions, then, as has been argued, there are serious consequences in relation to gender bias in how leadership behaviour and effectiveness is judged in the workplace. Areas affected include recruitment, appraisal, promotion, performance assessment practices and in processes adopted by organisations to identify and develop leadership potential. Certainly, in many countries, including the United Kingdom, senior positions in both the public and private sector are held predominantly by men (Table 13.2).

A review conducted by the Royal College of Physicians, entitled *Women and Medicine* (Elston, 2009), reported that by 2013 women will constitute the majority of GPs and by 2017 hospitals will also be dominated by female doctors. Currently, however, while forty percent of doctors are female, only twenty-eight per cent are consultants and of this population only seven per cent are consultant surgeons.

Table 13.2 Percentage of women holding senior positions in organisations in the United Kingdom in 2007/8.

Sector and organisation	Percentage of women
Public sector[a]	
Public appointments	34.4
Local authority chief executives	19.5
Health service chief executives	36.9
Senior ranks in the armed forces	0.4
Senior police officers	11.9
Senior judiciary (High Court judge and above)	9.6
Civil service top management	26.6
Chief executives of voluntary organisations	46.4
MPs	19.3
NHS consultants (all specialties)[b]	28.0
NHS consultants (surgeons)[b]	7.0
Private sector	
Board of directors of FTSE 100 companies[c]	12.0
Editors of national newspapers	13.0

[a]Public sector figures and percentage of editors of national newspapers based on data from Equality & Human Rights Commission, 2008.
[b]Data on women consultants is based on Elston, 2009.
[c]Data on percentage of females on boards of FTSE 100 companies from Cranfield University, 2009.

What type of leadership does a complex organisation need?

The 1980s and 1990s were dominated by models of 'visionary', 'charismatic' and 'inspirational' leadership, which emerged, in the main, from studies of senior and top leaders in large US corporations. However, the corporate scandals which led to the demise of organisations such as Enron, Amcom and WorldCom were attributed, in part, to the influence of these 'heroic' models. Growing concern was expressed about 'the dark side' of charisma, and the fact that some inspirational leaders can be not only obnoxious because of their self-aggrandising tendencies, arrogant and narcissistic but also dangerous, because their effect on organisations and employees can be very destructive (see Chapter 11). Some charismatic leaders can emasculate those around them and induce a state of 'corporate cultism' and over-dependence on themselves, or the one person at the top of the organisation. The term 'toxic leader' was coined in 1996 by US writer Marcia Whicker.

Heroic leadership is dead!

The challenges facing organisations, and particularly large public sector organisations such as the NHS where advances in medical technology incur greater expenditure, are growing in complexity, but at the same time available government funding is being reduced. There is a realisation that organisations need 'to do more with less' but without damaging staff morale and well-being, and that this will require the exercise of leadership at all levels, rather than relying purely on those at the top. Furthermore, organisations need to reflect the diversity of the communities they serve. This means that women and people from a variety of ethnic backgrounds should be represented at all levels, including the most senior.

The crucial importance of employee 'engagement'

The new focus for leadership is on how to increase employee engagement. Engagement has been defined as *an attitude*: having a strong positive attitude towards one's organisation and/or job; and *behaviourally*: displaying extraordinary efforts in applying oneself in one's job; but its essential characteristic is that a highly engaged individual exerts extra discretionary effort in what they do, which results in high levels of performance. There is substantial research showing strong associations between employee levels of engagement and their health and well-being, as well as a significant link between engagement and organisational performance, including recent studies in the NHS and other healthcare organisations (Table 13.3).

Case example: a new (inclusive) model of engaging leadership

Heroic models of leadership were based largely on focusing on 'distant', very senior, male leaders in US commercial organisations. But, to understand the nature of leadership that increases staff engagement in healthcare organisations, the methodology must

Table 13.3 Benefits of employee engagement.

For staff	For organisations
• Well-being, morale and health • Reduced depressive symptoms, somatic complaints and sleep disturbances • Reduced emotional exhaustion • Higher self-efficacy and commitment	• Customer satisfaction • Increased retention • Reduced absenteeism • Productivity • Profitability • Safety

focus on gathering data on bosses of various quality, and data based on the experiences of staff across the organisation with whom these bosses have worked. Any model must also be based on a truly inclusive sample of staff, that is by gender, level, ethnic background, age, occupational group, etc. One example of a model of engaging leadership emerged from a three-year study conducted in the NHS, involving a sample of over 2000 staff, and later extended and validated across the wider public, and private, sector. The model (Figure 13.1) comprises 14 dimensions of leadership behaviour. These have been described as four clusters:

- personal qualities and values;
- engaging individuals;
- engaging teams/the organisation;
- working in partnership with a range of different stakeholders.

This model of engaging leadership is essentially feminine in tenor, and resembles notions of 'servant leadership' with its emphasis on selfless actions that recognise and appreciate the contributions of others, and empower them to use their initiative and by so doing

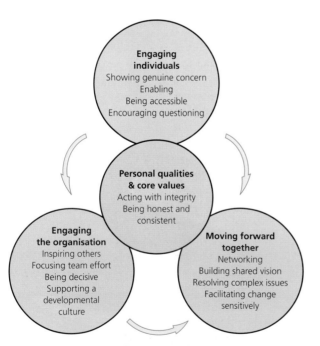

Figure 13.1 A new gender-inclusive model of engaging leadership. *Source:* Alimo-Metcalfe & Alban-Metcalfe, 2008.

become more effective as leaders in their own right. It focuses on strengthening relations with others, including members of one's own team, those being served, such as patients, carers, colleagues and partners in other organisations. It encourages questioning the status quo, judicious experimentation and innovation, and focuses on building shared visions and values and working in partnership, co-owning and co-designing the means by which change will be implemented.

Model's validity for predicting the motivation, morale and well-being of staff

A 360-feedback validated instrument based on this model, Transformational Leadership Questionnaire (TLQ), assesses the behaviour of individuals on the 14 dimensions, and includes items that assess 'leadership impact' on staff motivation, job satisfaction, commitment, reduced stress, etc. Table 13.4 displays a summary of the results of a discriminant function analysis of the 14 leadership scales assessed by the TLQ and their impact on staff motivation, morale and well-being from a sample of 5110 NHS staff (direct reports) rating their manager anonymously.

Model's validity for predicting the productivity, morale and well-being of teams

Leadership has to be embedded in the culture of organisations and teams to sustain its beneficial effects. A recent three-year longitudinal study funded by the Department of Health applying the TLQ to over 40 multi-professional teams in the NHS, controlling for a range of contextual variables, found that it predicted team productivity and morale and well-being. Box 13.2 describes the culture of highly engaged, high-performing teams.

> Box 13.2 **The culture of high-performing teams**
>
> - Feeling empowered by being trusted to take decisions
> - Feeling actively supported in developing one's strengths
> - Believing people are willing to listen to one's ideas
> - Time being made for staff to discuss problems and issues, despite the busy schedule
> - Feeling all staff were involved in developing the vision
> - Feeling involved in determining how to achieve the vision
> - High use of face-to-face contact

Leadership and team working in surgical teams

The rapid progress of medical research will necessitate creating cultures within teams of clinicians in which judicious experimentation and learning from mistakes will be of critical importance. A US study based on observations of 669 heart operations in 16 different hospitals investigated the characteristics of surgical teams

Table 13.4 Predictive relationship between the ratings of managers on the TLQ scales and their impact on staff.

	Job satisfaction	Motivation	Commitment	Achievement	Self-confidence	Reduced stress
Showing genuine concern	X	X	X	X	X	X
Being accessible	X	X		X		X
Enabling	X	X	X	X	X	X
Encouraging questioning	X			X		X
Inspiring others	X	X	X	X	X	X
Focusing team effort			X		X	X
Being decisive				X	X	
Supporting a developmental culture	X	X	X	X	X	X
Building shared vision	X	X		X	X	X
Networking	X	X	X	X		X
Resolving complex issues			X			
Facilitating change sensitively	X				X	
Acting with integrity			X		X	
Being honest and consistent	X	X	X	X	X	X

$N = 5110$ staff/managers

NB. This summary is based on discriminant function analysis of the TLQ dimensions on 6 of the leadership impact measures. While each of the TLQ scales is significantly correlated with each of the impact measures ($p < 0.01$), this figure shows relationships that are 'unique', i.e. cannot be accounted for by the other relationships.

that successfully adopted new micro-surgical techniques (Edmundson *et al.*, 2001). It found that what differentiated the 'successful' from the 'unsuccessful' implementers of the techniques were not factors such as the educational background, experience or status of the lead surgeon, but the fact that he or she 'gave up their dictatorial authority so that they could function as partners in the operating teams'. Such an approach is wholly consistent with the more feminine engaging style of leadership.

Are there gender differences in 'engaging leadership'?

Significant gender differences have been found in relation to how senior female and male managers/leaders in the NHS – some of whom were clinicians – were rated anonymously by their staff in the TLQ 360 process. Female leaders were rated as significantly more engaging than male leaders, irrespective of the sex of the person rating them. A study based purely on clinicians has yet to be conducted; however, these findings are consistent with separate research on the nature of patient–doctor communication.

Gender and doctor–patient interaction

The way clinicians react to patient information is determined to some degree by doctor–patient gender effects; research shows that female doctors remember more patient cues, especially in relation to history presentation and especially among women. Further, although there are male doctors with good communication skills, female doctors are seen to be better at breaking bad news to patients, using more patient-centred communication techniques and being more likely to make empathy-building statements. Female clinicians have been found to be more likely to engage patients as active partners and to offer emotional support as well as engaging in

psychological discussion, all of which have been associated with improved health outcomes.

Will having more women in senior positions increase engagement?

To assume that increasing the number of women in medicine will lead to an increase in the number of women in senior positions, and thus increase the chances of strengthening a culture of engagement in healthcare organisations, ignores the fact that, in many countries, organisational and career structures relating to medicine are themselves gendered. Choices of specialism are strongly gendered. Northern European studies have found fewer women entering surgical specialities, and tending to concentrate on a few specialties regarded as family-friendly, for instance those in primary care. Even though women now outnumber men in most medical schools, part-time working to accommodate child-care responsibilities still affects the career prospects for female clinicians, and for men who wish to share these responsibilities. Interestingly, in NHS management, women currently occupy 59% of all managerial positions (NHS Confederation, 2009).

While significant differences have been found in relation to gender and leadership style, the sex of the individual is itself no guarantee of particular forms of leadership and an engaging style can be developed by men as well as women, but some aspects of traditional male gender roles have been associated with a norm of a restricted expression of emotions. This limitation of expression, especially of emotions regarded as traditionally 'feminine', may be associated with a more managerial, or 'transactional', style of leadership rather than a style which is more engaging in nature.

In order to fully utilise the potential that exists within healthcare organisations, as with any organisation, there is a need to create a more engaging culture, but research and experience show that several organisational practices will need to be changed before this becomes a reality. Box 13.3 lists some of these.

> ### Box 13.3 Organisational practices that will support the creation of an engaging culture
>
> - Ensuring that recruitment, selection and promotion criteria include behaviours and approaches that reflect an engaging, inclusive style
> - Training assessors in understanding the nature and importance of engagement, and engaging behaviours at all levels
> - Appointing senior managers/clinicians who adopt an engaging style of leadership
> - Placing more emphasis in appraisal reviews on the discussion of how staff have adopted an engaging style in their day-to-day relationships, and in how they approach problems, make decisions and achieve their objectives
> - Including aspects of engaging leadership in medical training programmes, and providing opportunities to practise the skills involved in various clinical situations
> - Encouraging managers and clinicians, especially those who are in senior posts, to undertake 360-feedback that uses an engaging leadership model, and being strongly committed to supporting their development post-feedback
> - Supporting leadership development initiatives, team-building skills and leading change in ways that adopt an engaging approach

What greater feminisation of leadership could do for healthcare

The breaking-down of masculine or transactional styles of leadership and a shift to an engaging approach will not only increase the equality of both female and male clinicians but also better serve patients. The greater presence of women in leadership roles should impact on changes to the structures, and person-centeredness, of medical care and the transformative effect of a more humane, healthier, collaborative, productive and safer culture.

References

Alimo-Metcalfe B, Alban-Metcalfe J. *Engaging Leadership: Creating Organisations that Maximise the Potential of their People.* CIPD, London. 2008.

Cranfield University. The Female FTSE Index & Report. 2009, http://www.som.cranfield.ac.uk/som/p3012/Research/Research-Centres/Centre-for-Women-Business-Leaders/Reports, accessed 22 July 2010.

Edmundson AC, Bohner R, Pisano GP. Speeding up team learning. *Harvard Business Review* 2001; **79**(9): 125–32.

Elston MA. *Women and Medicine: The Future.* Royal College of Physicians, London. 2009.

Equality and Human Rights Commission. *Sex & Power: Who Runs Britain in 2008?* HMSO, London. 2008.

NHS Confederation. Reforming leadership development … again. NHS Confederation, London. 2009, http://www.nhsconfed.org/Publications/Documents/Debate%20paper%20-%20Future%20of%20leadership.pdf, accessed 21 July 2010.

Whicker, ML. *Toxic Leaders: When Organizations Go Bad.* Greenwood Press, Westport, CN. 1996.

Further resources

Alimo-Metcalfe B. *Gender & Leadership: Glass Ceiling or Reinforced Concrete?* Observatoire de l'Administration Publique, Québec, Canada. 2007.

Alimo-Metcalfe B, Alban-Metcalfe J, Bradley M *et al.* The impact of engaging leadership on performance, attitudes to work and well-being at work: A longitudinal study. *Journal of Health Organizational Management* 2008; **22**: 586–98.

Schein EH. *Organizational Culture and Leadership*, 3rd edn. Jossey-Bass, London. 2004.

CHAPTER 14

Leading Ethically and with Integrity

Deborah Bowman

St George's, University of London, London, UK

OVERVIEW

- Ethical leadership is informed by both external guidance and an internal commitment to its practice
- The process of making a decision is just as important as the outcome
- The notion of the 'virtuous leader' provides a way of thinking about ethical leadership that focuses on consistent and positive ways of working, irrespective of the context
- Using specific competencies and considering the way in which a 'virtuous leader' would respond to a situation ensures that leadership is considered, accountable and demonstrates integrity

---

The best measure of a man's integrity isn't his income tax return. It's the zero adjust on his bathroom scale. (Arthur C. Clarke)

Introduction

Clinical leadership is complex and requires diverse skills, but it depends on ethical awareness. Moreover, it is insufficient merely to understand ethical leadership in the abstract; rather, an authentic commitment to its practice is required. This chapter argues that, whatever the context, the practice of ethical leadership always depends on a particular set of attributes or, to use the language of ethics, *virtues*. A case study is discussed to demonstrate what it means to be an ethical leader in practice.

What is ethical leadership?

Ethical leadership derives from both external sources and internal choices, each of which is considered below.

External guidance on ethical leadership

There is a bewildering array of material available for those seeking to understand leadership, with authors variably engaging with the notion of ethical leadership (see Chapter 3). Box 14.1 summarises how some influential approaches to leadership relate to ethical concepts.

ABC of Clinical Leadership, 1st edition.
Edited by Tim Swanwick and Judy McKimm. © 2011 Blackwell Publishing Ltd.

Box 14.1 Leadership approaches and engagement with ethical concepts

Servant leadership: focuses on what it means to serve, to be in a position of stewardship and to hold the trust of those whom one serves. Its ethical antecedents are altruism, care, selflessness, honesty and probity.

Value-led leadership: requires leaders and organisations to reflect on the normative values which shape their work. Its ethical antecedents are virtue ethics and deontological theories.

Transformational leadership: a future-focused approach to which development, improvement or change is integral, often with the emphasis on improvement via effective and functional relationships. Its ethical antecedents are the consequentialist approaches where moral worth is evaluated with reference to possible outcomes, combined with theories such as feminist and narrative ethics which emphasise the significance of relationships and human interaction in moral decision-making.

These perspectives contrast with a more functional approach to leadership concerned with maximising the best outcome for groups or populations, for example staff, clients, patients or other interested parties. Its ethical antecedent is utilitarianism, in which moral decisions are made according to which choice is likely to produce the greatest good for the greatest number.

Aside from theories and over-arching approaches to leadership, what guidance exists for the individual who wants to ensure that their leadership is ethical? The NHS Leadership Qualities Framework (NHS Institute for Innovation and Improvement, 2010) is a relevant and accessible analysis of clinical leadership and its practice and Box 14.2 shows the how the framework captures the ethical dimensions of leadership.

The mixture of values and behaviours in Box 14.2 encapsulate much of what it means to be an ethical leader. However, it omits a crucial aspect of ethical leadership in practice, namely *consistency* of approach. The list in Box 14.2 is necessary but not sufficient: these values and behaviours must be consistently applied. Trust depends on predictability and reliability. Ethical leadership is dependable. Fallible human beings are susceptible to stress and personal predilection. No leader can eliminate these human tendencies. However, rigorous attention to process is a sound response to individual foibles and systemic variables. Decisions and actions that are informed by a careful and conscious process of consideration of specific precepts is an ethical decision. Intuitive or ad hoc decisions may serendipitously result in positive outcomes, but are ethically flawed if they are not made with due regard to principles and process. Put simply, ethical leadership is deliberate and aware rather than accidental and inexplicable.

Box 14.2 External guidance on ethical leadership derived from the *NHS Leadership Qualities Framework*

- Prioritise patient interests and safety
- Respect for, and support of, others
- Awareness of self and impact on others
- Honesty and integrity
- Accountability and conscientiousness
- Team working and collaboration
- Commitment to service

Source: NHS Institute for Innovation and Improvement (2010).

The internal component of ethical leadership

Whilst leadership can be learned, truly ethical leadership requires internal reflection and personal commitment to a coherent set of core values. Being a virtuous leader depends on an individual's willingness to become self-aware, emotionally intelligent and reflective. Whilst theoretical models and development programmes can be helpful, without a genuine commitment to, and belief in, the ethical dimensions of leadership, credible and authentic leadership is unlikely (Gilbert, 2005). Without internal commitment to the virtues of ethical leadership, behaviour is likely to be dissonant, inconsistent or unpredictable, leading to inequity, unreliability or unfairness. The virtuous leader is not a return to 'trait'-based leadership, where individual characteristics are identified as more or less suitable for leadership. Rather, it is an approach that assumes everyone has the ability to become self-aware, to reflect critically, to adapt and develop their strengths and weaknesses, but acknowledges that such a process is lengthy, challenging and requires a commitment by those who are serious about becoming and remaining ethical leaders (Oakley & Cocking, 2008). Value-led leaders are willing to challenge others and to address conflict whilst advocating for better healthcare or improved patient safety (Shale, 2008).

The virtuous leader in practice

So what does ethical leadership look like in practice? Box 14.3 presents a short case study that considers virtue-based leadership and provides a structure for practice.

Mr Holmes and the anaesthetists: Discussion

The discussion outlines the principal ethical issues to be considered in relation to the list in Box 14.2.

Box 14.3 Case study: Mr Holmes and the anaesthetists

Mr Holmes is the clinical team lead for surgery and anaesthetics in a large tertiary referral centre. For some time, the anaesthetists have been concerned about staffing levels, especially as ambitious plans to develop two specialist surgical centres within a wide catchment area are being developed. The anaesthetists expressed their concerns informally to Mr Holmes, who was sympathetic and offered to discuss the situation with the Medical Director. The Medical Director listened carefully to the concerns but said he could offer no more staff or resources to the department. One Monday morning, Dr Mayes, a newly appointed consultant anaesthetist, comes to see Mr Holmes and tells him that a patient died on the table over the weekend. She believes that, although the patient was very sick, low staffing was also a factor. She explains that she was covering three theatres and in the end had to ring her specialist trainee to ask if he would come in 'as a favour' and help because she was so pressured. She asks Mr Holmes what he 'is going to do about this completely untenable situation'.

Prioritise patient safety and interests

The anaesthetists believe that patient care is compromised. Even if there is not a causative relationship between the patient death and staffing provision, Dr Mayes is seeking a response from Mr Holmes. There is, at the very least, a question about patient safety to be addressed. Information is crucial if progress is to be made: what are the actual effects of the levels of staffing? Mr Holmes spoke to the Medical Director previously, but there is an imperative to seek further detailed information about staffing in anaesthetics and its impact on service commitments. Information must be represented honestly to the Medical Director. If the Medical Director disagrees that patient safety is an issue, comprehensive and clear information will allow Mr Holmes to ask questions about the risks of current anaesthetic staffing in the context of plans for specialist surgical services. Using a carefully drawn account of the issue(s) makes explicit the moral problem and allows Mr Holmes to discuss specifically how existing provision and proposed change influence the common commitment to patient safety.

Respect for, and support of, others

Mr Holmes should inform staff what he is doing and why (which, of course, requires Mr Holmes himself to know what he is doing and why). He needs to support his team but avoid being seduced into false promises. If Mr Holmes makes a commitment, it must be met. Simple actions such as setting a timescale for making progress and informing the team of any meetings or decisions reflect a genuine respect for, and support of, others.

Similarly, Mr Holmes should act respectfully towards the Medical Director and listen to his perspective, engaging in constructive discussion rather than obdurate advocacy for 'his' team and patients. It is likely that everyone will, to some extent, have an emotional response, which must be acknowledged but not allowed to distort how the issue is addressed. Dr Mayes may be feeling angry, frightened, guilty and anxious following her experience and Mr Holmes should enable her to express her emotion and be supportive even as he is determining the next steps.

Everyone in an organisation has different roles and perceptions and there can be multiple versions of the 'truth' about a situation. Using the information he acquires as he investigates further, Mr Holmes should seek to influence with integrity and respect those who may see the situation differently, trying to understand difference where it occurs and using new information to revisit core issues.

Awareness of self and impact on others

Mr Holmes may have an intuitive response to Dr Mayes. It may be sympathy, a sense of solidarity, shared frustration, guilt that the experience happened to one of 'his' team, irritation ('another problem') or defensiveness. The history and hierarchy of their relationship is relevant too. It is essential that ethical leaders are aware of their own reactions to others: the colleague whom one finds 'difficult' or who has a 'reputation' must be treated as fairly as the colleague with whom one trained.

By being aware of the effect of relationships on his responses and taking time to reflect critically on what is revealed by an initial response, Mr Holmes is acting ethically. His is a considered, self-aware response that acknowledges human interaction and its inevitable effects on leadership.

Honesty and integrity

Mr Holmes must be scrupulously honest. All communications should be accurate. Honesty and integrity are essential to trust and credibility: there is much more at stake here than the specific question of staffing. Honesty and integrity require Mr Holmes to keep both Dr Mayes and the Medical Director informed. He must be open about what he is going to do and meet commitments. Exaggerated promises, omitted details and premature reassurance will compromise not only the resolution of this specific situation but also Mr Holmes's reputation and credibility, weakening him as a leader, perhaps irrevocably.

Accountability and conscientiousness

Ethical leaders respond in a timely way. Mr Holmes should make himself available to Dr Mayes. If, as is common in the NHS, there are competing priorities, Mr Holmes should explain when and how he expects to investigate Dr Mayes's concerns. Patient safety has been raised as a concern and a prompt response is indicated. At each stage, Mr Holmes should be open about his actions and the rationale for his proposals, and be prepared to respond professionally to challenge. Leadership requires effort, application and patience. An ethical leader understands the importance of adhering scrupulously to proper processes. Mr Holmes must see events through. However brilliant a leader may be in a crisis, routine or difficult situations must be addressed through to their conclusion. An ethical leader is

accountable and conscientious even when exciting new challenges beckon.

Team working and collaboration

Leaders depend on their teams and must work collaboratively across an organisation. Regrettably, situations can quickly degenerate into quasi-territorial disputes in which adversarial positions are assumed and unhealthy alliances dominate. Mr Holmes may be part of several teams (e.g. clinical teams, management teams, educational teams). Mr Holmes brings to each team a genuine commitment to collaboration in which imaginative solutions are sought, individual interests are seen as dependent on collective outcomes and quiet empowerment is preferred to charismatic direction. These actions will enable Mr Holmes to retain the support of his team long after the particular staffing issue is resolved.

Commitment to service

Service encapsulates the essence of ethical leadership, namely that committed, respectful, inclusive, person-centred practice is its primary function. Yet individualism is still often actively encouraged and promoted in medicine and it can feel challenging to subjugate personal interests to those of others, even when to do so is a professional obligation. Feelings of frustration, irritation or even resentment may emerge. Indeed, one could argue that to deny such feelings is misleading and ultimately unhelpful in seeking to develop and maintain leadership. The key is to acknowledge the human variables, biases, intuitions, assumptions and values that all leaders have, whilst simultaneously understanding that such feelings must not influence behaviour and diminish the integrity of leadership (Pendleton & King, 2002).

Mr Holmes may reflect on the core purpose of healthcare and his role to elucidate what it means to serve. It is a simple, but powerful, step in articulating what is often assumed and throws into sharp relief the 'bottom line' of an individual's obligations. Merely by asking 'What does it mean to serve in this situation?' and 'What do we actually mean by patient safety?' Mr Holmes is beginning to demonstrate his commitment to service.

Conclusion

This chapter has argued that there are both external and internal factors that shape what it means to be an ethical leader. Statements of standards, staff development and consistently applied processes are integral to ethical leadership. However, the role models that are visible within, and provide leadership of, an organisation are the most powerful tool in ensuring that ethical leadership is valued, enacted and maintained. As Albert Einstein observed, 'setting an example is not the main way of influencing another, it is the only way'.

Finally, when all or most parties are in agreement about what should be done and this is in accordance with core values and patients' rights, leading in such contexts is fairly straightforward. However, clinical leaders are often required to make decisions where there are no clear or 'right' answers, when (because of limited resources or other issues) the best that can be done is a compromise. This causes a conflict between what our ethical stance, 'moral compass' and core values would suggest as the way forward and what is actually possible in any given circumstances. This is where the real challenges for value-led leadership lie.

References

Gilbert P. *Leadership: Being Effective and Remaining Human*. Russell House Publishing Ltd, Lyme Regis. 2005.

NHS Institute for Innovation and Improvement. NHS Leadership Qualities Framework. 2010, http://www.nhsleadershipqualities.nhs.uk/assets/x/50131, accessed 22 July 2010.

Oakley J, Cocking D. *Virtue Ethics and Professional Roles*. Cambridge University Press, Cambridge. 2008.

Pendleton D, King J. Values and leadership. *British Medical Journal* 2002; **325**(7376): 1352–5.

Shale S. Managing the conflict between individual needs and group interests: Ethical leadership in health care organizations. *Keio Journal of Medicine* 2008; **57**(1): 37–44.

CHAPTER 15

Developing Leadership at All Levels

Judy Butler

Coalescence Consulting Ltd, Bath, UK

OVERVIEW

- Leadership development should not take place in a vacuum: there needs to be a compelling reason understood by all

- It is important to be clear on the knowledge, skills and behaviours to be developed and what successful demonstration will look and feel like

- Applying an understanding of how people learn will ensure that the most appropriate development solutions are adopted in the right sequence

- Considering the timing of leadership development is critically important

- Good leadership is developed through a variety of means, including an extended period of exploration, practice, feedback and reflection

- The support of leadership development in the workplace is crucial

Introduction

Leadership development is more likely to succeed when a number of underlying factors are considered and managed. These include

- a compelling reason for the learning;
- knowing how success will look and feel;
- appreciating how individuals prefer to learn;
- early opportunities to apply learning;
- ongoing feedback and support.

We have a compelling reason.

'Making change actually happen takes leadership. It is central to our expectations of the healthcare professionals of tomorrow' (Darzi, 2008). This quote from a key UK policy document is just one of many that could have been selected to show the increasing importance placed on encouraging clinicians at all levels to consider their leadership role.

In health systems across the world clinicians are needed who understand the nature of leadership and themselves have a well developed set of capabilities to apply at any time and are prepared to take on leading clinical and managerial positions and responsibilities. The challenge is in enabling the development of those capabilities in a timely and consistent fashion so that they may be demonstrated in any of the many situations described earlier in this book and contribute to the performance of individuals, their teams and the organisation.

In this chapter we will explore

- how competency frameworks may support the identification and development of good leadership;
- how an understanding of learning preferences can help in selecting from and sequencing different types of development support;
- when leadership development should be addressed so that it is a supported and cumulative process;
- how to ensure newly acquired skills, knowledge and behaviours are sustained over time.

Using competency frameworks

There are a growing number of leadership competency frameworks across the public sector, including the recent *Medical Leadership Competency Framework* established by the Academy of Medical Royal Colleges and the NHS Institute for Innovation and Improvement (2010). Organisations may also articulate their own sets of competencies, describing leadership in a language that reflects their particular culture. Typically, these contribute to an annual appraisal cycle, but can also be used to support recruitment and ongoing development.

The primary aim of a framework is to clarify the main areas of capability required at a given time either for a specific role or for an overall topic, such as leadership. It should be answering the question 'What will make the difference between effective and ineffective performance?' Each capability area is broken down into clearly defined skills, knowledge and behaviours in order that they can be more readily observed, assessed and developed.

Competencies can be written to reflect different levels of capability, aligned to different levels in organisations, as shown in Table 15.1. This allows individuals to understand and seek to develop those needed to progress or to operate more successfully in increasingly complex situations and roles. For example what leadership is a newly qualified consultant required to demonstrate?

ABC of Clinical Leadership, 1st edition.
Edited by Tim Swanwick and Judy McKimm. © 2011 Blackwell Publishing Ltd.

Table 15.1 Competency frameworks: a worked example.

Competency area		Impact and influence	
Brief description		Persuades, convinces and gains the respect and agreement of others	
Level	*Definition*	*Indicators may include*	*Negative indicators may include*
Level 1	Confidently explains own views when questioned and refers to, or quickly accesses, relevant factual information	• When questioned can refer to, or quickly access, relevant factual information • Gives an accurate picture of the situation	• Lacks confidence and withdraws from discussions when questioned
Level 2	Tailors own approach, taking account of the audience and their requirements	• Adapts the content, style and tone of presentations/discussions to appeal to others' interests • Anticipates and prepares for others' reactions and plans how to tackle objections	• Does not understand the needs/interest of the audience and therefore is unable to gain buy in
Level 3	Uses own personal network across departments to enable him/her to keep up to date with views and feelings to obtain a range of perspectives on organisational issues	• Successfully influences at all levels to strengthen own case • Builds trust with clinical partners, colleagues, peers • Confronts areas of non-performance for mutual benefit	• Takes a low-key approach and is not perceived by others as having presence

Increasingly, those behaviours that limit an individual's perceived or actual capability are also included. These can support discussion on why an individual is not being as effective or successful as desired. See Table 15.1 for a worked example.

Used well, competency frameworks provide insights into the behaviours and approaches that are valued. They support the feedback process by encouraging a conversation around key areas, inform personal development plans and clarify routes to different roles and levels. However, there are some notes of caution:

• It is difficult to write simple, unambiguous statements of behaviour that reflect the overall capability sought.
• The resulting lists of skills and personal attributes may be overwhelming and appear unachievable.
• An underlying assumption of most frameworks is that leadership resides in a single individual, whereas contemporary notions of distributed leadership argue for leadership as an embedded characteristic of organisations.

Selecting the right development activity

Individuals like to learn in different ways. Although this may simply be an expression of personality, Honey and Mumford (1982) argue for four distinct learning styles. Each preferred style lends itself to different development opportunities. For example, *Activists* are more likely to respond well to on-the-job experience, or to programmes that provide role-play exercises and business simulations. *Reflectors* are more likely to select action learning sets, and benefit from coaching, mentoring or shadowing. *Pragmatists* also respond well to business simulations, but need them to reflect how they see their world and to be allowed to implement their learning soon after. *Theorists* respond to the opportunity to read around a subject in advance, to debate and test the intellectual basis.

In reality, the ideal learning environment will require individuals to operate in each of the four styles so that new knowledge, skills and behaviours are truly embedded through a sequence of experience, reflection, application and experimentation (Kolb, 1984). Understanding preferred learning styles shows where best to start so that the individual is engaged early in the process, and where additional support may be required to maintain momentum later. Some of the more common approaches to leadership development are reviewed below.

Coaching and mentoring

Coaching and mentoring sit on a spectrum of learning relationships that enable individuals to take charge of their own development. Each activity is built around a conversation which aims to release the potential of the 'client', or 'mentee', and to help them achieve results which they themselves value. The terms *mentoring* and *coaching* are often used interchangeably but have some generally agreed distinguishing characteristics.

Coaching provides the opportunity to reflect upon and develop knowledge, understanding and skills through a series of one-to-one conversations. It is distinct from both counselling (the coach is not there to give advice) and from mentoring (on which more in a moment). Coaching is usually short term, bounded and revolves around specific development areas or issues. The coach is not required to have any specific contextual knowledge. Over several months of regular meetings, the coach will use a series of questions to help an individual think through a situation: past, present or future to help them:

• challenge their own assumptions;
• consider differing perspectives on a single issue or event;
• set a goal and work out the best approach;
• look ahead at the potential barriers and risks.

To get the most from coaching, individuals should

• have a clear goal;
• be prepared to own both the issue and the solution;
• not seek a ready answer – it won't be given.

Coaching can be expensive and therefore frequently reserved for more senior individuals. This is not necessary and it is possible to develop good coaching skills within an organisation or system, making it more affordable at all levels.

Mentoring has a different flavour. The relationship here is usually more long term, with a general remit of aiding the mentee's overall professional development. The role of a mentor is to provide the mentee with an insight into a different or new environment, to make links and open doors. Mentoring is often used to enable new employees to understand more about the culture and the 'way things are done', to give access to networks and the opportunity to experience situations outside their day-to-day work. It is an ideal mechanism for clinicians wanting to know more about the management side of the NHS. And, as with coaching, open-minded mentors find they learn almost as much as the mentee.

Shadowing

Shadowing is a much undervalued activity. In a system as complex as the NHS, a frequent complaint is that one part of the system doesn't understand another part. Shadowing gives the opportunity to observe and learn without being required to act. It is an aid to understanding rather than skill development but, for the pragmatists, it can be a good incentive to subsequently develop a new set of approaches. Like mentoring, shadowing also provides opportunities for role-modelling, a rich source of many forms of social learning (Kenny *et al.*, 2003).

Action learning sets

Action learning sets are being more commonly used within broader development programmes. Frequently combined with master classes, they provide individuals with opportunities for reflective practice based on the concepts explored in the master class. Groups of 8–10 people work together on real issues to support each other to understand and plan how to take situations forward.

They work equally well with individuals from within one, or across several, organisations. However, there must be a common thread between them, either in type of role, seniority or in a common goal. They are not expensive to set up but do need to be maintained as the relationships and trust needed within the group take time to develop.

Masterclasses

These large group events provide all levels with opportunity to consider a new topic, stimulate new ideas and thinking or to be re-energised on an old topic. They do not support in-depth skill development but, as with the shadowing, they may stimulate an interest for further development later.

Formal development programmes

Finally, there are the broad training programmes that often lead to academic credits or a postgraduate qualification. They are usually conducted in multiple modules spread over a number of weeks or months. This is a vibrant and growing market and careful selection in line with a clear aim is important.

The benefits include:

- a balance of academic rigour and experiential learning;
- time to apply new concepts between modules and revisit progress in a managed environment;
- the opportunity to learn from and with those from different work environments.

However, such programmes may be expensive and time-consuming and sometimes the appeal of a further academic qualification can outweigh the real value of such a programme to an individual's career.

Feedback

Introducing new knowledge, skills and behaviours and providing an opportunity for practice is not enough. When developing any interpersonal behaviours – and leadership sits firmly in this category – multiple perspectives on style and approach are vitally important as they reflect the reality of being a leader interacting with a range of people and within different situations. Feedback

Table 15.2 Guidelines for successful feedback.

Giving feedback	Receiving feedback
Check what feedback is wanted	Say what areas you want feedback on
Be specific, use examples	Listen carefully
Focus on behaviours that can be changed	Use questions to clarify and check you have understood
Balance positive and negative aspects	Take time to sort out what you have heard
Check you have been understood	Look for trends when getting multiple perspectives

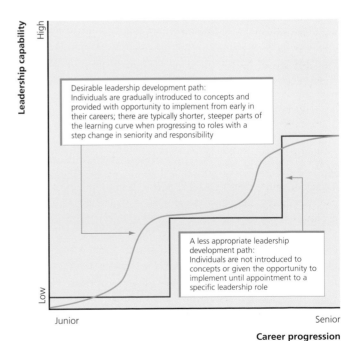

Figure 15.1 Timely development. Source: Dr Fiona Moss, with acknowledgement.

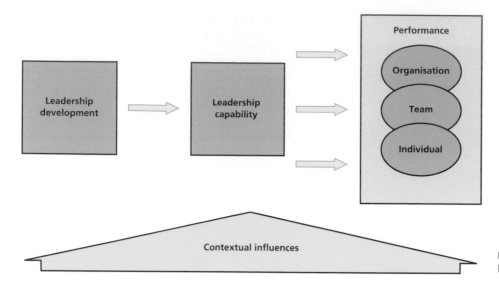

Figure 15.2 The relationship between leadership development and performance.

is an essential part of the learning process and by identifying the trends in the feedback and separating out the extremes there is more opportunity to identify and develop the approaches that will more usually succeed. The quality of the feedback and the way it is transmitted and received is key to maximising its powerful development potential. Table 15.2 provides some simple guidelines for giving and receiving feedback.

A number of formal mechanisms exist for feedback in the form of multi-source instruments. The NHS Leadership Qualities Framework 360 is a good example (NHS Institute for Innovation and Improvement, 2010).

Timely development

In many public sector organisations, leadership concepts and the opportunity to develop the capabilities of an effective leader are not consistently introduced until the point at which a leadership role (such as service line head or clinical director) is taken on. Until then, learning is focused on clinical expertise and little time is spent understanding the broader picture or the capabilities needed to navigate it successfully for oneself or for a team. Figure 15.1 compares a desirable path (green) with that usually experienced by clinicians (blue).

Timely development is not just a question of starting earlier. As with any new set of capabilities, it is about ensuring that individuals can take a cumulative approach, considering basic concepts early on and having the opportunity to put them into practice at that time.

Leadership development and performance

The answer to the question 'Does leadership development work?' is a complex one. Based on a growing evidence base, there appears to be a positive correlation between leadership development and the performance of individuals, groups and organisations. But the relationship is complex and the causal links between development strategies, such as those described above, leadership capability and enhanced performance are poorly understood (Figure 15.2). There is much still to learn and understand, but effective leadership development appears to be about bringing together a series of interventions in a timely and consistent fashion. It depends on the understanding and openness of the participant to learning new behaviours; it depends on the authenticity and integrity of the different types of programme selected; and, mostly, it depends on a consistent level of support available back at work (Box 15.1).

Box 15.1 **Case study: Fellowships in clinical leadership**

As one component of a London-wide strategy of leadership development, NHS London and the London Deanery devised the 'Darzi' Fellowships in Clinical Leadership. This innovative programme provides a cohort of trainee doctors with a unique opportunity to develop the organisational and leadership capabilities necessary for their future roles as consultants and clinical leaders. 'Darzi' Fellows are appointed across primary, acute, foundation and mental health trusts. The posts comprise 12 months 'out of programme' from specialty training, during which time Fellows work on a number of projects covering service change, quality and safety improvement and leadership capacity building, under the guidance of a nominated medical or clinical director. The Fellows are supported throughout by a leadership development programme, including coaching, project consultancy and taught sessions leading to the acquisition of a postgraduate certificate.

References

Darzi A. *A High Quality Workforce: NHS Next Stage Review*. Department of Health, London. 2008.

Honey P, Mumford A. *The Manual of Learning Styles*. Peter Honey Publications, Maidenhead. 1982.

Kenny N, Mann K, MacLeod H. Role modeling in physician formation: Reconsidering an essential but untapped educational strategy. *Academic Medicine* 2003; **78**: 1203–10.

Kolb D. *Experiential Learning: Experience as the Source of Learning and Development*. Prentice Hall, Englewood Cliffs, NJ. 1984.

NHS Institute for Innovation and Improvement. NHS Leadership Qualities Framework. 2010, http://www.nhsleadershipqualities.nhs.uk/assets/x/50131, accessed 22 July 2010.

Further resources

Bolden R. *What is Leadership? Leadership South West Research Report*. Centre for Leadership Studies, University of Exeter, Exeter. 2004.

Connor M, Pakora J. *Coaching and Mentoring at Work: Developing Effective Practice*. McGraw-Hill, Maidenhead. 2007.

NHS Institute Board Level Development. Coaching. 2010, http://www.institute.nhs.uk/building_capability/general/executive_coaching.html, accessed 20 July 2010.

NHS Institute for Innovation and Improvement. Medical Leadership Competency Framework. 2010, http://www.institute.nhs.uk/assessment_tool/general/medical_leadership_competency_framework_-_homepage.html, accessed 20 July 2010.

Pedler M, Burgoyne J, Boydell T. *A Manager's Guide to Leadership*. McGraw-Hill Professional, Maidenhead. 2004.

Index

CURRENT TITLES

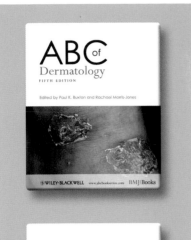

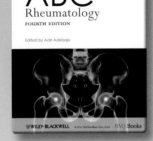

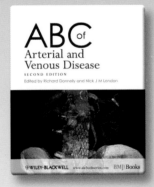

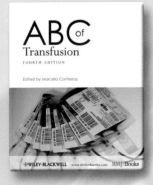

ABC of Dermatology
5TH EDITION

Edited by Paul K. Buxton & Rachael Morris-Jones
Consultant Dermatologist, Hampshire; King's College Hospital, London

- A new 20th anniversary edition of this bestselling *ABC* covering the diagnosis and treatment of skin conditions for the non-dermatologist
- Covers the core knowledge on therapy, management and diagnosis of common conditions and highlights the evidence base
- Provides clear learning outcomes and basic science boxes
- Includes a new chapter on the general principles of skin condition management for specialist nurses

March 2009 | 9781405170659 | 224 pages
£28.99/US$52.95/€35.90/AU$57.95

ABC of Rheumatology
4TH EDITION

Edited by Ade Adebajo
University of Sheffield

- A practical guide to the diagnosis and treatment of rheumatology for the non-specialist
- Fully revised and updated to include information on new treatments and therapies while covering the core knowledge on therapy, management and diagnosis
- A highly illustrated, informative and practical source of knowledge offering links to further information and resources
- This established *ABC* is an accessible reference for all primary care health professionals

October 2009 | 9781405170680 | 192 pages
£27.99/US$44.95/€34.90/AU$57.95

ABC of Arterial and Venous Disease
2ND EDITION

Edited by Richard Donnelly & Nick J.M. London
University of Nottingham; University of Leicester

- A practical guide to the diagnosis and treatment of arterial and venous disease for the non-specialist, focusing on the modern day management of patients
- Explains the different interventions for arterial and venous disease
- Covers the core knowledge on therapy, management and diagnosis and highlights the evidence base on varicose veins, diabetes, blood clots, stroke and TIA and use of stents
- This revised new edition now includes information on new treatments and therapies, antithrombotic therapy, and non-invasive techniques

April 2009 | 9781405178891 | 120 pages
£26.99/US$49.95/€33.90/AU$54.95

ABC of Transfusion
4TH EDITION

Edited by Marcela Contreras
Royal Free and University College Hospitals Medical School, London

- A comprehensive and highly regarded guide to all the practical aspects of blood transfusion
- This new edition is an established reference from a leading centre in transfusion
- Includes five new chapters on variant CJD, stem cell transplantation, immunotherapy, blood matching and appropriate use of transfusion
- Reflects the latest developments in blood transfusion management

March 2009 | 9781405156462 | 128 pages
£26.99/US$49.95/€33.90/AU$54.95

For more information on any of the titles, please visit the *ABC* website at **www.abcbookseries.com**

ABC of Mental Health
2ND EDITION

Edited by Teifion Davies & Tom Craig
Both King's College, London Institute of
Psychiatry

- Provides clear practical advice on how to
  recognise, diagnose and manage mental
  disorders successfully and safely

- Includes sections on selecting drugs and
  psychological treatments, and improving
  compliance

- Contains information on the major
  categories of mental health disorders, the
  mental health needs of vulnerable groups
  (such as the elderly, children, homeless
  and ethnic minorities) and psychological
  treatments

- Covers the mental health needs of special
  groups: equips GPs and hospital doctors
  with all the information they need for the
  day to day management of patients with
  mental health problems

May 2009 | 9780727916396 | 128 pages
£27.99/US$47.95/€34.90/AU$57.95

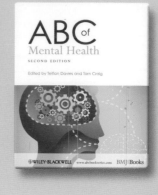

ABC of Lung Cancer

**Edited by Ian Hunt, Martin M. Muers &
Tom Treasure**
Guy's Hospital, London; Leeds General
Infirmary; Guy's & St. Thomas' Hospital,
London

- A practical guide for those involved in the
  care of the lung cancer patient

- An up-to-date evidence-based review of
  one of the most common cancers in the
  western world

- Written by the specialists involved in
  the launch of the NICE UK Lung Cancer
  Guidelines

- Looks at the epidemiology and diagnosis
  of lung cancer, focusing particularly on
  primary care issues

April 2009 | 9781405146524 | 64 pages
£21.99/US$37.95/€27.90/AU$44.95

ABC of Spinal Disorders

**Edited by Andrew Clarke, Alwyn Jones,
Michael O'Malley & Robert McLaren**
Royal Devon and Exeter Hospital; University of
Wales Hospital, Cardiff; Warrington Hospital;
GP

- This brand new title addresses the causes
  and management of the different spinal
  conditions presenting in general practice

- Provides much needed practical guidance
  on the diagnosis, treatment and advice as
  back pain is one of the commonest causes
  for absence from work and is a chronic
  problem confronting general practitioners

- Includes guidance for the GP when they
  have to refer patients for more specialist
  treatment

December 2009 | 9781405170697 | 72 pages
£19.99/US$35.95/€24.90/AU$39.95

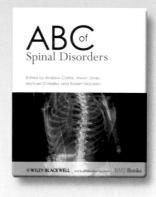

ABC of Medical Law

**Lorraine Corfield, Ingrid Granne &
William Latimer-Sayer**
Guy's and St Thomas' NHS Trust, London;
University of Oxford; Lawyer, Clinical
Negligence and Personal Injury Specialist

- Fills the gap for a basic introduction to
  legal issues in health care that is easy to
  understand and act upon

- Provides up to date coverage of
  contentious issues such as withholding and
  withdrawing treatment and confidentiality

- Accessible to those without any legal
  knowledge, providing guidance without
  becoming embroiled in complicated legal
  discussion

June 2009 | 9781405176286 | 64 pages
£19.99/US$35.95/€24.90/AU$39.95

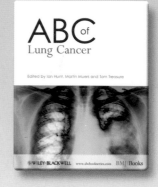

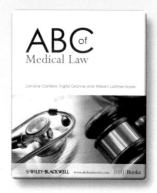